THE FIVE STAGES
OF
~~DEATH AND DYING~~
Getting well

Judy Edwards Allen, Ph.D.

LifeTime Publishing

Library of Congress Catalog Number: 92-073490
ISBN 0-9627954-0-2

The author gratefully acknowledges permission to reprint excerpts from the following published materials:

A Course in Miracles
© Copyright 1975
Foundation for Inner Peace, Inc.

The Song of Prayer: Prayer, Forgiveness, Healing
© Copyright 1978
Foundation for Inner Peace, Inc.

Getting Well Again
© Copyright 1978
O. Carl Simonton and Stephanie Matthews-Simonton

Goodbye to Guilt
© Copyright 1985
Gerald G. Jampolsky, M.D.

Love, Medicine, and Miracles
© Copyright 1986
B. H. Siegel, S. Korman, and A. Schiff

LifeTime Publishing
6663 SW Beaverton-Hillsdale Highway, Suite 166
Portland, Oregon 97225

Acknowledgements

With gratitude and love to my family, who saw my perfection even when I couldn't, to my doctors and nurses, to my friends and colleagues—all who participated in my healing. I will not name them all here. They know.

Some names have been changed to protect the truly innocent.

"This picture of me...never suffered pain at all. It witnesses to the eternal truth that [we] cannot be hurt, and points beyond itself to both your innocence and mine. ...see that every scar is healed, and every tear is wiped away in laughter and in love. ...look on our forgiveness there, and with healed eyes...look beyond it to the innocence...that is the proof that we have never sinned."

A Course in Miracles Text p. 526 (First edition)

Table of Contents

"For some have entertained angels unaware."

Hebrews 13:2

To my angels:

my mother Frances Reed
and my husband Jack Allen

Prologue

The Cancer Carousel

---

*I*n the autumn of 1979, just before I turned forty, I discovered a walnut-sized lump in my right breast. It was, of course, cancer. "Of course," because in the year previous to that discovery my career had taken a disheartening and humiliating nose dive. My husband had begun an affair with my boss's wife and I was too depressed to acknowledge it. My last child had left home—a kind of freedom I had looked forward to for years but now found to be an awful wrench.

Why *not* cancer? Why *not* me?

A year earlier I had been on top of the world—at the peak of an exciting career, satisfying marriage, children turning out well, and in perfect health. Suddenly it all caved in. Cancer was simply a bleak and final demonstration of the hopeless situation I felt myself to be in.

I had surgery, a simple lumpectomy with no follow-up treatment. It seemed a minor event in view of the collapse of my marriage. As I began to put my life back together as a single woman, I felt that cancer was behind me. I found I had an inner strength that could overcome disaster and depression. My career revived and I bought new, wild and colorful clothes to celebrate the bonus of weight loss without dieting. I didn't need a prosthesis since only about a quarter of my breast had been removed. I had hit bottom and I rebounded with a new joy and aliveness that I hadn't felt for a while.

A contented year passed, and I fell in love unexpectedly with a widower, a long-time friend and colleague. Our wedding in the spring of 1981 was an event of celebration and delight, the signal for me that life was normal again. My attention now centered on the fulfillment of my personal life rather than on my job.

The regular out-of-town travel and the pace and pressure of my career, which had been a pleasure for so many years, was becoming a source of strain and irritation more often than gratification. I was ready for a career change, a slowing down, with less emphasis on prestige, money, and success. I no longer needed those affirmations. Their achieve-

2

ment had not held the promised fulfillment. Still I stayed on the job, noticing I was tired more and more of the time but unable to see any good alternatives. I began to search for a less stressful job.

Three years after the first cancer a second growth appeared. Six months of anxiety passed while doctors continued to assure me there was nothing there. Finally surgery confirmed a major recurrence, a metastasis of breast cancer behind the chest wall. This new tumor, I was told, left me with little hope of survival. My oncologist predicted another metastasis within three months, and no hope of survival after that. He would go along with radiation but he was against chemotherapy, believing it to be pointless in my case.

I got second and third opinions, desperate for some hope but finding none. The consulting oncologists both agreed on followup treatment—six weeks of daily radiation, then chemotherapy.

I found a new oncologist who recommended at least three years of chemotherapy—it was clear he expected it to continue until my death.

Thus began my ride on the cancer carousel. Once on board, it seems one has little choice but to ride in endless circles, knowing the music will stop soon and it will all be over. Doctors and nurses counseled me to "Get out of denial, dear." Apparently Elisabeth Kubler-Ross' five stages of death and dying—denial being stage one—would be part of this ride, and the patient is expected to be sensible and obedient in passing through those stages in an orderly fashion.

I began the treatments. I obeyed doctors' orders. I certainly experienced some of the other stages of dying—anger, bargaining, depression—but not acceptance.

It was while fighting this alarming recurrence and the effects of treatment that I began seriously to search for my spiritual resources. It was an undertaking unlike anything I had worked at in the past. It was deadly serious. Life or death. Medicine did not hold any hope for me, and I had to find alternatives to that. This book is a story of that time, told in part by excerpts from my journal, and it is a story of ultimate triumph.

Chemotherapy ended after nearly two years, early in 1985. Over the months of treatment the dosage had been gradually decreased as my blood cells lost their ability to withstand the toxicity. Finally the treatment seemed to be doing more harm than good, and we stopped. I was told that I would almost certainly have another recurrence of cancer within just a few months. Three months, most likely, if the probabilities derived from research were to be trusted.

Seven months later, in August of 1985, my radiation oncologist and my surgeon each independently found another small tumor in the same place as the first one. This was the recurrence they had been expecting, and they weren't happy about it but they weren't surprised about it, either.

This time, having discovered immense spiritual resources that I believe to be available to everyone who seeks such help, I decided to refuse the recommended medical interventions, at least for a while. Clearly, the medical treatments had not worked. I wanted to give my own treatment a chance. Ignoring my doctors' anxiety and their strong objections, I turned myself over to my higher Self for healing.

4

That was seven years ago. The tumor was gone by September of that year, and the intervening month was for me a movement at Hyperwarp speed into the truth about healing. I will try to tell you about the stages of healing that I went through, and what I have discovered so far. I don't believe now that there are necessarily five stages. There may be thirteen, or two. In fact, there may be only one truly essential stage, and that is the final one—acceptance.

For most of us, however, going through all the preliminary struggles to get to the final healing seems to be necessary. When I arrived at what I thought was the final stage, I discovered it to be the first stage of something undreamed of—life from a healed mind. And this is where I have no words to describe it.

Everyone must find, as I did, their own particular way to heal. My experience may give some clues, some signposts. My specific truth may not be true for others. Others may use different words for similar concepts. I am convinced now, however, that all of us have within ourselves the power to heal.

The inner power to heal has been documented by hundreds of studies. Locke and Rowan at Harvard University have summarized 1300 research projects demonstrating the connection between mind and the immune system, the bedrock of our own healing power. In the new medical science of psychoneuroimmunology (the study of the interrelation of mind/emotions/immune system), carefully designed studies are beginning to produce measurements of the effect of mind and emotions on the actual number of disease-fighting cells.

Medical science may never be able to put the final touch of proof on what appears finally to be a matter of the human spirit. Many medical practitioners may question the evidence of healing that I and so many others have reported. Spontaneous remission is not understood, and when cancer patients recover in spite of a death sentence, medical scientists are willing to credit only the medical therapy the patient has received. "Chemotherapy won't help," my oncologist told me in 1983, but in 1985 it had changed to "Chemotherapy must have done it."

Stages

I had not given much thought to death the first time I had cancer. It was easily treated, I thought, by surgery. But when the second cancer was found, death suddenly loomed large and imminent. I had heard of the five stages of death and dying from helpful medical professionals, and now set out to understand what they were. I was in denial, and it was clear that I was expected to move on to the next stage, and the next, and to begin to prepare for the final stage: acceptance of my impending death.

Try as I might, I could not move out of denial. Denial seemed to me to be the only sane and sensible way to deal with a death sentence. Were these five stages the only alternative I was to be offered? Was death the only possible outcome? I denied it, and continued to deny it. I read Elisabeth

Kubler-Ross' book *On Death and Dying,* and realized that I was stuck in stage one.

While I was stuck there, I began to formulate a different set of stages, with a different outcome: healing. I got well, in spite of the doctors' negative predictions. Others asked me for help in dealing with their own cancer, and I began to write a book about the five stages of getting well. Before I got very far with the book, doctors found the third cancer.

During the succeeding weeks of intense inner work, the fifth stage became clear to me for the first time. It was the same as Kubler-Ross' final stage: acceptance, but with a unique twist. Permanent healing is, first, healing of the mind—spiritual healing. Healing of the body may follow, and often does. But, even if physical healing has not occurred, to die with a healed mind is a happy death.

The Five Stages of Dying

Dr. Elisabeth Kubler-Ross is an unusual physician, a pioneer in the field of death and dying. She has taken death out of the closet by observing that death is as much a part of life as is birth, and should be acknowledged and prepared for. She observed that dying people often went through certain predictable stages, sometimes in great mental and emotional distress. The people around them, including doctors and nurses, were unable to help. Families and medical helpers felt helpless to cope with the non-medical aspects of dying.

With her workshops and lectures and books Kubler-Ross gradually got some of the reluctant doctors to listen. "Quit lying to your patients," she demanded. "Tell them they are dying. Recognize and cope with the emotional fallout that facing that reality will create for them."

From her experience with dying patients, Kubler-Ross described five stages that patients go through between diagnosis and death. The stages are not necessarily experienced in sequence, and the patient may encounter a stage more than once, or get stuck in one of the stages. I recognized several of the stages from my own experience.

Denial is the first stage. "This can't be true. I am going to get better," says the patient, in the face of a terminal diagnosis.

Then, Kubler-Ross maintains, the patient stops denying and gets mad. The focus for the anger is frequently the doctor who delivered the bad news. Or it might be a family member, or God, or Fate, or everyone within range.

Anger and rage yield to bargaining. (God, if you just let me live I'll volunteer as a counselor in a camp for children who have cancer. I'll jog every day. I'll become a vegetarian. I'll even go to church.)

Bargaining gives way to depression. Each of these stages, Kubler-Ross' observes, can last from days to months. Depression is the next-to-last stage. All else has failed. God Himself has abandoned the dying person. Silence reigns. Tears. Introspection and withdrawal, and grief.

The fifth and final stage is acceptance. This is the time when family members notice the patient's growing detachment, peace and calmness. Then,

Death comes soon, padding softly on foam slippers, and leaves the survivors with a sense of awe rather than horror.

Understanding these stages can ease the suffering of those who are dying, and of those who love them. Yet, there can be an alternative.

The Five Stages of Getting Well

Five stages of getting well, in counterpoint to the five stages of dying, slowly became clear to me as I went through them. I observed similar stages in talking to others who were getting well, and read about the same patterns in stories of people who recover from cancer. I gave names to the stages and tried to pay attention to their characteristics, so I could tell others about them. The rest of this book is about those stages, and some positive techniques to use in experiencing them. You may discover that for you there are more or fewer than five stages. Nevertheless, the techniques can be used as part of of your own personal survival kit.

Stage One:
Denial of the Negative Prognosis

The first stage in getting well is to make a deliberate, conscious choice to live. Stage one is the same one identified by Kubler-Ross, denial. But it is a rejection, not of the *diagnosis* (cancer, and it is serious), but rather a denial or rejection of the *prognosis* (you're probably going to die). To put it in more positive terms, it is a conscious decision to get well and to live, rather than to die. It may feel at first as if you have no choice in this matter, that Fate has taken over and decided for you. Not so. You get to choose.

Stage Two:
Taking Charge of Your Treatment

Stage two is deciding to take charge of your treatment. One of the worst things about cancer is the overwhelming feeling that your body has betrayed you, that you are out of control, at the mercy of the whirling carousel of cancer tests and treatments. The treatment may seem worse than the disease at times. But you can be in control of your medical treatment. You can and should take charge of all that happens to you.

Stage Three:
Taking Charge of Your Lifestyle

Stage three is a challenge to be tackled once your medical treatment has been decided upon and is under way. In stage three you will take charge of your lifestyle. The role of stress and conflict in the onset of cancer seems to be clear. While it may seem that some conflict cannot be avoided, you can choose to eliminate some of the sources of stress in your life. It may require, as it did in my case, dramatic lifestyle changes.

Stage Four:
Taking Charge of Your Attitudes

Even more important than changing your lifestyle is changing your mind. Stage four is taking charge of your attitudes. Although there is controversy about whether or not there is a "cancer personality," some research seems to indicate a relationship between state of mind and cancer. You may not be able to change your lifestyle or to eliminate stress but you *can* control how you react to it. We have just begun to understand—and accept— the power of the human mind. We use only a tiny fraction of the power of our minds, and too often we turn its power against ourselves, destroying our own health and happiness when we could be creating wellness and wholeness instead.

Stage Five: Accepting Your Healing

The final stage in getting well has been the most difficult for me to understand and to carry out. It is, again, similar to Kubler-Ross' final stage: acceptance. Now, however, you are not asked to accept your impending death but simply to let go and accept your healing. Having taken charge of your treatment, changed your lifestyle and your attitudes, and found the creative energy of the life force, it is hard to learn to then relinquish control, turn yourself over to the grace of a higher power and let all that you have set in motion carry you to its logical conclusion: wholeness of mind, body and spirit. Wellness.

You can choose. The five stages of dying can be eased if they are understood, and you can choose to begin those stages. It is the most highly personal choice you will ever make and there should be no blame or guilt attached to the decision. Or you can choose to wait a while and to begin instead the five stages of getting well. It's up to you.

Chapter One

First Stage:
Denial of the Negative Prognosis

Climbing on My Carousel

---

*W*hen a close friend learned that her mammogram had shown a suspicious area she was most distressed about, as she put it, "climbing on the cancer carousel." Tests, X-rays, bone scans, blood tests, biopsies, surgery, radiation, chemotherapy, quarterly checkups, more mammograms—it seemed that once she placed herself in the hands of the cancer establishment, her life was never free of such routines again, even if she got well.

My turn came in mid-August, 1979. It had not been a good day—in fact, it had not been a good year. When the high-profile job in Alaska went bad we moved back to Oregon where I spent brooding hours wondering how much to blame myself, and having black fantasies of revenge against the person in Alaska I preferred to blame instead. My life had developed all the elements of the most wretched soap opera: the other woman was not only my husband Bruce's new business partner, but was my boss's wife—and she lived next door.

Saturday, August 18, was the day of our friend Carleen's marriage. At the last minute Bruce backed out of going to the wedding, once again choosing to spend the day working in the upstairs bedroom with his partner Mary.

I left the house quickly, took Bruce's new red Volvo—Mary's color choice—and popped the clutch on my way out, spraying gravel on her lawn.

The wedding was lovely, sweet, a ceremony of love and laughter and joy, and a knife in the heart to me. I had lost all love and laughter and joy, could barely remember those emotions. I had not been fun to live with, as Bruce put it, for many months. I stayed at the wedding as long as I could, putting off going home until it was dinnertime. I would have to go home for dinner. Mary would have to go home for dinner.

Rebellion gripped me and I didn't go home. Let him fix his own dinner. Let him eat alone, as I so often did. I didn't call. I always called if I would be late for a meal but this time I drove around the city instead, noticing how deserted it was on a Saturday night; stopped for coffee; killed time. There was nowhere to go, nothing to do. I considered the public library, and decided that would be just too desperate. Finally at ten o'clock I drove home. I walked in the front door casually, cooly ignoring Bruce's questioning look. He said he'd been worried. I shrugged. He acted guilty, contrite. About what?

He was asleep as soon as we went to bed, while I sat up reading a magazine. As I turned a page, a headline grabbed my attention:

DES Mothers at Greater Risk for Breast Cancer

DES headlines always caught my eye. Nineteen years earlier when I was pregnant with my daughter, a doctor gave me diethylstilbestrol, a hormone commonly prescribed in those days to prevent miscarriage. Years later it was found to cause vaginal cancer in girl children born of mothers who took the drug. Moreover, it was found to be useless in preventing miscarriage. My daughter had vaginal adenosis, a precancerous condition of the cervix. I didn't miss many DES headlines.

I had not examined my breasts for some months. I lifted my fingers to my right breast and there it was: a well-defined, hard lump the size of a walnut. My breath stopped. How long had this been there? How could I have missed it?

The next morning was Sunday. On the way to the airport for a business trip to Honolulu Bruce and I stopped at the emergency room. The doctor on duty brushed aside my fears, assuring me it was a cyst. "Nine out of ten of these lumps are just cysts. It's probably nothing. Get a mammogram."

Three days later, back from Hawaii, I called for a mammogram appointment. It would be four more

15

days before they could fit me in. I didn't argue. This news could wait.

After the mammogram I started to worry in earnest. How would I hear the results? Would someone call? How would I get in to see a surgeon? Would I need a surgeon?

My annual appointment for a blood pressure check was already scheduled for two days later. I called the nurse and asked her to have the internist get the mammogram and interpret it for me. He would.

I sat on the table in the paper gown, shivering from air conditioning and anxiety. The internist I had seen at least once a year for the last several years appeared in the doorway, his toes just over the threshhold. He held my chart and the mammogram results in his hand.

"You wanted the results of the mammogram?" he asked.

"Yes, please," I said.

"Well, it's inconclusive," the doctor told me. "There's too much dysplasia to see anything. You'll have to see a surgeon."

I knew about getting an appointment in this organization. It was always "six weeks." I needed one *now*. "Will you make an appointment for me?" I pleaded.

"No," he replied. "You can do it yourself. Just call. They'll get you in."

"I've never had that kind of luck. Will you at least recommend a surgeon? You know them, don't you? Why can't you call for me? I don't even know who to call." I was groveling.

"You just call for an appointment, and if you have any trouble getting in soon, let me know and

I'll see what I can do. You won't have any trouble." He turned and left the threshhold.

Our appointment was over. He had not checked my blood pressure—he had not even come into the room. Surely he couldn't be so busy he would ignore the original reason for the appointment—could he be afraid of cancer?

I went to the pay phone in the lobby and dialed the appointment center. "We can get you in early in October," was the crisp response to my request for an appointment with a surgeon—any surgeon.

"But you don't understand," I persisted. "I have a breast lump, and the mammogram is inconclusive—I have to see a surgeon right away."

She left the line. Minutes later she came back, trying to be helpful. "Well, we can schedule you for September nineteenth, no sooner."

She didn't respond to my protests. That was the best she could do. It was now August 27.

I hurried back to my internist's office, and explained to the nurse that I needed to talk to him again. He had promised he would help me get an appointment with a surgeon if I couldn't get one, and I couldn't get one. The nurse was unable to help me. He had just left on a two-week vacation.

Back to the pay phone. I took September nineteenth.

At work I found Carleen, just back from her honeymoon. She had had breast cancer a year earlier and was treated in the same health maintenance organization. She adored her surgeon, and was happy with the treatment she received. I asked for her help and she was quick to respond. Her surgeon's nurse was now a friend of hers, someone Carleen could call and explain the situation. The nurse, compassionate and understanding, made an appointment for me with Carleen's surgeon for August 30.

I liked Dr. York immediately. He was kind, gentle. He decided that there was no way to identify the lump as a cyst without a needle biopsy—inserting a hollow needle into the lump and drawing out fluid. The fluid would then be tested for malignant cells. If there were none, it was a cyst. He was quick and deft with the needle, and it was over quickly. He gave me a pat and said reassuringly, "Nine out of ten of these things are cysts. There's probably nothing to worry about."

Bruce and Mary were away on a business trip. I went next door to find Mary's husband Dave and his son Mark, a medical resident. They were in the kitchen cooking dinner. Apparently they had already heard about the lump. I asked Mark what he thought it might be.

"Is it hard?" he asked.

"Yes," I said.

"Is it fixed, or movable?"

"Fixed."

"Oh," Mark replied.

"Well, what does that mean?"

"Oh, it's just hard to say. It could be anything," Mark said. "It's probably nothing."

He kept his face impassive and incommunicative. But as I turned away, I caught the look he flashed at his father. Mark's mother, Dave's first wife, had died of breast cancer eight years earlier after a series of surgeries. I remembered seeing her the last year she was alive, when she came to office parties. She sat in a rocker, not speaking, not moving except for flashing knitting needles, weak and small and wasting away.

I went to the bookstore and bought a new book my mother had mentioned to me a few months earlier, a revolutionary book about treating cancer with psychotherapy and positive visualization. Just in case. *Getting Well Again*, by the Simontons in Houston, provided convincing data about how imagery and visualization, along with positive expectations about the outcome, can contribute to survival. I read the whole book in one sitting and decided to start by having positive expectations about the biopsy. In fact, my expectations were so positive that I stopped worrying and decided that it was indeed just a cyst. I wouldn't need to use imagery and visualization because I didn't have cancer. I would simply expect a happy outcome.

Positive expectations helped the next week pass more comfortably, and I completed plans for a vacation trip to California with my three teenage children. It would be just the four of us. The kids were all at the age where they were establishing their own lives, and this would likely be the last time we would be together in such a way. Their stepfather Bruce had not shared vacations with us for the last year or two, and did not want to come this time either.

I rented a large R.V. to try out a new mode of travel. My daughters Kelley and Lauric came home from college the day before our departure date of September sixth and together we packed the R.V. full of food, games, jigsaw puzzles, books, and tapes. We would pick up Mike, the oldest, at the university on our way south.

On Thursday, September sixth, we were in the R.V. ready to leave when I remembered something and ran back into the house. The telephone was ringing. I answered it against my better judgment

—I had left the motor running. It was the chief of surgery at the hospital. Dr. York was on vacation. The needle biopsy of the "probably nothing" lump had revealed that it was malignant. I was to come in immediately to arrange for surgery the following week.

Kelley and Laurie moved in close and stayed close during those first few awful hours. They went with me to the clinic to schedule surgery and have further tests—chest X-ray, bone scan. (Had it already spread?) I was assigned to Dr. Fisher, who explained to me that he would do a partial mastectomy—a lumpectomy—which would preserve most of the breast and was as safe as complete breast removal. He strode back and forth across his office.

"If you're going to insist on a total mastectomy, you'll have to go to some other hospital," he told me. "I won't do one in a case like yours. I don't believe it's necessary."

He had a belligerent, feisty manner which I liked. I'd go along with his recommendations. I trusted him. He called the oncologist, Dr. Davidson, and made an appointment for me for the next day. The carousel had begun to spin, and I was on it.

That evening I paced in front of the house, restless, needing air. Dave drove by, home from work. He stopped the car in the middle of the street and I walked over to his window. No words, just his warm hands covering my cold hands on the car windowsill in silent, sympathetic support. He had expected this. He understood. It helped.

Friday I saw Dr. Davidson. He examined me, supported the partial mastectomy recommendation, and told me about his research study. He was an investigator in a national long-term study to

20

determine the effectiveness of partial mastectomy with or without followup treatment as opposed to complete breast removal with or without followup treatment.

Dr. Davidson assured me that there was no indication that radiation and/or chemotherapy were necessary after surgery. He told me that as far as anyone knew for sure, partial mastectomy with no followup was as effective in eliminating breast cancer as was a radical mastectomy with radiation and chemotherapy. They needed subjects for the study. Would I participate?

I agreed, since I would be in the "no followup" group and he assured me that was the treatment he would have recommended in any case. No risk, then. I was relieved. Radiation scared me, and I had refused dental X-rays for years. Radiation causes cancer. Everyone knows that.

I asked Dr. Davidson about the Simontons' theories. He chuckled. "If you want to mess around with that stuff, you'll have to go talk to the ladies in the back." He jerked a thumb back toward the building behind the clinic, a house remodeled into office space for the ladies in the back, two counselors who helped cancer patients deal with the psychological effects of diagnosis, prognosis and treatment.

I didn't go to the ladies in the back—instead I used the pay phone in the lobby to make an appointment for the following Monday, the day before surgery, with a psychiatrist Carleen recommended. If I was going to find out how my personality or lifestyle might have contributed to the development of a cancer, I might as well start now. I had begun doing intense positive visualization for an hour, twice a day. I visualized the

21

cancer as weak and helpless, as the Simontons suggested in their book, and saw my own white cells as strong and aggressive in destroying them. I visualized myself as strong and healthy—and victorious over cancer.

Both Dr. Fisher and Dr. Davidson felt a hard lump under my arm, and predicted that there would be lymph node involvement. I'd been reading, so I knew what that meant. The malignancy had spread to my lymph system, and from there would likely spread throughout my body. If it turned out there was lymph node involvement, I would be taken out of the research study and given chemotherapy.

I decided not to accept that possibility. My visualizations and imagery began to focus on a small localized tumor. I told both doctors I thought they were wrong, and that there would be no lymph node involvement. They smiled, humored me, bided their time.

Friday night Bruce came home from his business trip. It was late, and he had not expected to find me there. But the R.V. still loomed in the driveway, obviously not on its way to California. He opened the door and stopped, putting down his bags. Why hadn't I left? I told him the diagnosis and the schedule, feeling a little triumphant—let Mary demand that he stay uninvolved in this!

One should always ask, when one is ill, three questions:

- • • What was going on in my life when the illness started?
- • • Whom do I need to forgive?
- • • What did the illness buy me?

I didn't ask these questions, because I had only begun to be aware of the powerful effect of the mind and emotions on the body. I hoped that this obviously serious illness would bring Bruce to my side, providing comfort and support and love, and send Mary packing.

That Friday night as Bruce sat and absorbed the bad news in silence, I suggested that we all use the prepaid R.V. to go to the beach and have a fun weekend, instead of moping around the house. He declined to join us. Clearly, this illness was not going to buy me a thing.

Mike arrived on the bus and we had a lovely weekend, a time-out with the kids, flying kites on the beach, playing games and playing house in the R.V. It renewed my spirit for the week ahead.

The psychiatrist on Monday wasted little time on the cancer diagnosis. He got right to the heart of the matter: my husband was bailing out of the marriage. Until then I had not admitted it out loud to anyone, not even myself.

Surgery Tuesday morning. Afterward I was euphoric, buoyed up by the outpouring of love, roses, cards, visits, stuffed animals and phone calls from people I hadn't realized cared for me that much. Except from Bruce. He visited occasionally, but observed that I had more than enough flowers from other people. Once I was on my feet Mike, Kelley and Laurie returned to college.

Saturday, the day before I was to leave the hospital, Bruce told me he was leaving on a business trip that night with Mary. I didn't protest. I was beginning to collect injustices, beginning to feel martyred.

Saturday night I lay in a nearly empty hospital and felt utterly alone. Visiting hours were over. I could see the lights of the city and imagined that everyone but me was happy and had a loving partner. Just as I was working myself into a full-blown depression Carleen sneaked past the nurse on duty to bring me dangly bright earrings she had made herself, and a loving card. She stayed long enough for me to feel comforted.

Sunday I was discharged from the hospital. I hadn't planned ahead for this. Sitting on the bed fully dressed, I wondered how I would get home. I didn't want to call a friend and have to explain that Bruce was gone. I had no money with me, so couldn't take a taxi. I swung my legs and brooded.

While I sat immobilized my sister and her husband bounced in, in town to visit me and delighted to be able to take me home. Later that night Carleen appeared at my house, bringing good cheer and exotic tropical juices to promote quick healing. I wasn't alone after all—until she left and the empty house fell still and quiet.

I needed reassurance before I could fall asleep and called Bruce in Alaska. Once again I hoped that he would recognize and respond to my need for emotional support. Instead he was angry with me for sounding needy. (Or with himself for feeling guilty?) From the way he sounded on the phone I was certain that Mary was in his room.

How many more signs would I need to verify that our marriage was over? The illness left me incapacitated emotionally as well as physically, and I was unable to take any action at all to repair the marriage or to end it. It limped on and I grew more despairing, stopped at every turn by my own apparent fragility.

I looked for apartment ads in the Classifieds, then realized I couldn't yet physically handle the packing and moving. If I asked him to move out, then I would have to see him arrive every day to pick up Mary next door. I wanted out, but felt paralyzed. I had told no one but my psychiatrist of the affair, which Bruce still insisted was my paranoid imagination. I often believed it was just that, no longer trusting my intuition or even the accumulating, damning evidence.

My Death Wish

Five weeks after surgery I drove my car into an unmarked intersection and was struck broadside by a truck I didn't see coming but which had the right-of-way. I awoke in the ambulance on the way to the hospital I had so recently left. A concussion, broken teeth and a broken rib now added to my miseries. I wasn't surprised. I was beginning to recognize my own death wish.

My first real confrontation with that unconscious death wish came a week after the accident. I had driven myself to the clinic (Bruce and Mary were out of town) for a marathon session with doctors. First I saw an internist about the broken rib which was painfully located just under the incision. Next was a neurologist about the effects of the concussion—I still had headaches, trouble walking and focusing my eyes, and a black eye made even uglier by the blood-red eyeball. Worst of all—since I made my living with my brain—my brain seemed to have gone on an extended vacation.

The last doctor I saw that day was the surgeon. The mastectomy incision was not healing properly and the breast remained red, swollen and painfully filled with fluid. Every week Dr. Fisher drained it with a large needle. By the time I found myself lying on the surgeon's examining table, I was feeling desolate.

Dr. Fisher examined the festering flesh with concern. "You know," he said, "this just isn't normal. I'm afraid the cancer may have come back. You wait right here [so I was planning to go somewhere?] while I get my knife. I'm going to do a biopsy."

He left the room and shut the door. I lay under the sheet, stretched out like a bug on a pin, drowned in a feeling of utter aloneness and helplessness. I debated the options for a moment. What I most wanted to do was to throw myself on the floor for a real kicking, thrashing, bawling two-year-old tantrum. I wanted to refuse to go along with the program. I wanted to run naked and shrieking through the waiting room and out the front door, trailing my sheet. I wanted to lose control. I wanted *out*. I hit bottom.

It took the doctor a long time to get his instruments. Instead of throwing myself on the floor I closed my eyes and tried to quiet myself. Yes, I was alone. I had driven myself to the clinic, and would drive myself home. There had been no support from my husband, nor would there be. The marriage was over, had been over before I got sick. If I was so determined to die I would have to do it alone.

In the end we all die alone anyway, even when surrounded by loving family. Dying is the most intimate, personal, private thing we can ever do.

But did that mean I was not only alone but also helpless?

No.

Slowly, an image of myself took shape in my mind: my body was hollow, and inside me was a smooth white ceramic cylinder—like the nose cone of a space ship. Heat, friction or abuse cannot mar the perfection of the ceramic. It is perfectly flawless, invulnerable and impenetrable. Indestructible.

That image gave me great comfort and peace. It seemed to represent the truth about me. Where did it come from? At that point I didn't know or care. I had survived, I was still intact. I would continue to survive. Whatever part of me was trying to kill me would not win this battle. The biopsy was endured, and five days later came back negative. I started, finally, to heal.

That desolate moment of utter despair after the first cancer was the moment when I decided to deny death, to live instead of die. The decision, although not entirely a conscious one, nevertheless represented an important turning point for me.

Denying Death

"Refusal to hope is nothing more than a decision to die."
Bernie Siegel, M.D.

Dr. Bernard Siegel, a surgeon and professor of surgery at Yale Medical School, has written an extraordinary book which should be required reading for cancer patients, and for doctors who treat cancer patients. The book, *Love, Medicine and Miracles*, describes Dr. Siegel's "lessons learned about self-healing from a surgeon's experience with exceptional patients." He has observed that fifteen to twenty percent of his cancer patients consciously or unconsciously wish to die and accept the diagnosis as a way out of a life that has become unendurable. Another sixty to seventy percent perform to satisfy the physician. They do what they're told to do, and trust in the medical treatment to cure them.

The other fifteen to twenty percent are exceptional patients. They refuse to play the victim, want to participate in every aspect of their treatment, question everything, reject negative prognoses.

Bernie Seigel asks his patients four questions in addition to the medical history:

1. "Do you want to live to be a hundred?"

The capacity to be an exceptional patient is accurately predicted by an immediate, visceral "Yes!" with no ifs, ands, or buts. "Yes" means "I feel in control and enjoy living."

2. "What does this disease mean to you?"

If the patient thinks cancer means death the patient has a problem. So does the doctor, if he is prepared to deal with the patient's beliefs about cancer.

3. "Why did you need the illness?" (that is, "What does it buy you?")

4. "What happened in the year or two before you became sick?"

These questions reveal Siegel's belief that the causes of cancer, and the reasons why some get well and some die, may not yet be explainable by science alone.

The answers to these questions can tell the doctor more about the patient's chances of recovery than the medical history. A patient who does not want to live to be a hundred probably does not want to live until next year, in her deepest heart.

Stage one in getting well is the denial of the negative prognosis, the denial of your own unconscious death wish, and the conscious and deliberate decision to live.

If you don't want to live, cancer may be as good a way as any to die, and better than most. It involves less guilt and blame than suicide. It may even be better than a sudden lethal heart attack. There is time to reap a harvest of love, time to say good-bye to everyone; time, perhaps, to forgive and be forgiven; time to be comforted; time, even, to know in advance the truth of the phrase we all mutter at times—"They'll be sorry when I'm dead."

It may be that you have already made a decision to die and a cancer diagnosis is simply the manifestation of that decision. Though the decision may be unconscious, it need not be final. Cancer gives you the opportunity to recognize that a decision has been made, and to reconsider. Now the decision can be made at the *conscious* level, to live or to die.

You may not know whether you want to live or die. Cancer is a clue. There are some ways to find out. Ask yourself Bernie Siegel's questions. Do you want to live to be one hundred? Do you want to live another ten years? Five?

Raise your arms straight out to the sides, parallel to the floor. Have someone watch while you say loudly three times, "I want to live!" If your arms begin to drop while you are making this statement, your unconscious mind may be telling you it does not agree with what your mouth is saying.

A friend newly diagnosed with cancer was asked by her doctor to do this exercise while he watched. As soon as she spoke the words "I want to live," her arms began to drop. At the same time she realized with a shock but with clear certainty that her words were not true. She had no idea that deep inside she had decided she wanted to die. Now that her wish had been made visible she had to face it. Her life was filled with trauma and anguish and she was tired of the struggle. She felt depressed and hopeless.

Yet, once confronted, my friend found that she could regain her will to live. She struggled with the unconscious death wish now made conscious, and she eventually made a conscious choice to fight for her life, and she got well.

Think about your future. Can you see it clearly? Do you have plans beyond next year? Are you looking forward to it? Do you have things you need to finish? Even if you can't see your future, do you know it's there?

Early in my talks with the psychiatrist he asked me what kind of future I saw for myself. With his question, I recognized that I no longer had a vision of what life might hold for me beyond the day I was living right now. My task then was to rebuild my vision of my own future, and to want to participate in living in that future.

It may take some time for you to be able to know whether or not you wish to live or to die. It's not socially acceptable to want to die, even if you are very old, very sick, or very weary; even if life is no longer rewarding. Cancer may be a socially acceptable way out, but you may not want or be able to admit that perhaps you choose it.

Choosing to die is okay. It's honest, and realistic for some people. Dying is inevitable in any case. The only choice you really are making is one of timing. If you decide that in fact your usefulness is over and you do not want to live longer, that should be respected and allowed. You may find that you have to fight your loved ones harder for the right to die than you would have fought the cancer. But you get to choose your own fight.

The choices are all yours. You will present your body for the surgery, the radiant rays, or the chemotherapy drugs. If you're lucky, a loved one or two will be nearby, giving support with words and touches. But you will have a moment early in the process when you confront the future with utter clarity, knowing how lonely and important is your role in this drama.

You may reject the idea that it is even possible to make a conscious choice to live or to die of cancer or some other disease. You may believe that your own unconscious destructive force cannot be challenged. You may believe in an unkind fate, karma, and randomness. You may believe that God punishes His children by giving them cancer and makes them suffer for their sins. Doctors may give you poor odds for your survival.

If you decide to live you will have to challenge all of those beliefs. You may have to challenge your doctors. It will take stamina and persistence and hard work. But you will be in charge of all that happens to you, and you will have become an exceptional patient.

Death is not the swift and certain outcome of cancer. That is a truth that is difficult to accept, given the beliefs of society, of our friends, and most importantly, of our doctors.

Doctors believe in cancer and they believe in death, because they see so much of it. People who get well when they weren't expected to don't go back to see their doctors. If they do go back, the doctor decides that his diagnosis was wrong, or that the treatment that was only intended to be palliative was responsible for a cure instead. People who get well in spite of medical predictions aren't discussed in the medical literature. Self-induced healing is considered too mystical to report in the journals.

Try to imagine being an oncologist and treating cancer patients day after day, only twenty percent of whom genuinely want to fight to live. It would be difficult to believe in the power of the human mind and spirit to conquer an illness—particularly if all of your training had been focused on scientific and technological solutions to disease. How disheartening it must be to know that the best you can offer a patient is treatment that in itself is debilitating and destructive. Doctors who stay in such a profession deserve our gratitude and our compassion, and can certainly learn from us.

I go back to see my oncologist for regular checkups—not because I still fear a cancer relapse, but because I want him to see me, again and again, as a reminder that he has collaborated in some success stories.

After diagnosis of the second cancer I saw Dr. Boles for a second opinion. Several knowledgeable friends had told me he was the best oncologist in Portland. My physician friend, Mark, told me Dr. Boles was the most aggressive oncologist he knew, unwilling to give up on a patient to the very end. Shortly after I spent an hour discussing my own case with Dr. Boles, I read a full-page feature article in *The Oregonian* entitled "It Only Hurts When They Die," subtitled "Doctors discuss dealing with the failure when technology, talent can't save patients."

Dr. Boles was quoted extensively in this article. He discussed his excruciating pain when he lost a patient. I know he suffered in these cases, for my daughter-in-law was a nurse in his hospital and had seen him cry with the family when a patient died. For an oncologist like himself, he added, "you accept from the outset you're going to lose."

This is the deeply held belief of the doctor who is known as the best in town and the most aggressive in fighting cancer. Reluctant to let go of the patient, reluctant to lose—yet his expectation from the outset is that he *will* lose, that his patient will die.

Cancer often kills, and most of us know about that. Oncologists certainly know about it. We've all heard the horror stories. But the truth is, you don't have to die of cancer. You don't have to accept the beliefs of the rest of the world, or of your doctors. Miracles of healing are far more common than we realize, since they are not reported in the research literature, in magazines or newspapers. They don't show up in the obituaries.

It may be that the *prognosis*—a forecast of the probable course of the disease—kills, rather than the cancer itself. Having been told and retold your chances, it is difficult not to accept the prognosis as inevitable.

Shortly after seeing Dr. Boles for the second opinion I heard a radio news story about a child with cancer, and a phrase used by the newscaster rang in my ears: "The doctors have given him six months to live." What a prognosis. How difficult it is to resist and deny such authoritative words. I doubt that doctors ever actually say, "I give you six months to live." It's a cliche, but one with terrible power to set up a self-fulfilling prophecy. Why do we use such words to rephrase what the doctors actually *have* said to us about statistical probabilities? What a gift. Six months to live. No hope.

If you decide to live you must reject a negative prognosis. You must do it now. You must refuse to internalize anything anyone says to you about limits to your chances of getting well and staying well. Dying of cancer becomes a self-fulfilling prophecy, a belief that perpetuates and fulfills itself. If you start willingly moving through the stages of death, you will of course arrive at the final stage, acceptance, and then you will probably die.

Acceptance of your approaching death, in fact, may be the first stage of dying.

Denial is the first stage of getting well.

The Will to Live

In a book that has been reprinted fifteen times since its first publication in 1951, Arnold Hutschnecker, M.D., explained scientifically the interconnection of the human psyche and the body. *The Will to Live* has become a classic, helping many people to reduce their anxiety and fear, encouraging them to attempt to recognize and to resolve their inner conflicts by themselves. The chapter "Man Dies When He Wants to Die" for the first time discussed death openly, allowing people to overcome their desperate fear of dying and to come to terms with death as a natural part of living.

In his book Hutschnecker revives Freud's concept that within each of us rages a constant battle between the will to live and the will to die—his explanation for suicide. He discusses case histories of apparently healthy people who suffer from constant anxiety about their health—a whisper of danger from the unconscious. Whether the danger is real or imagined, the threat to health is real. Freud's concept described only two basic instincts, Eros, which is love or the creative instinct, and Thanatos (named for the Greek God of Death), the destructive instinct, or the death instinct.

How these two opposing drives function in each individual, for harmony or disharmony, health or sickness, long life or early death, for the fullness of living or the poverty of it, Hutschnecker points out, depends upon the individual. He further shocks us by quoting Karl Menninger who believed that we determine not only our end but the means by which we die. As Menninger stated it, "In the end each man kills himself in his own selected way, fast or slow, soon or late."[1]

My father believed the Bible literally, and expected to die when he had reached three score years and ten. Accordingly, shortly after his seventieth birthday he was diagnosed as having colon polyps that were almost certain to be malignant. Surgery followed, to remove the polyps and confirm the diagnosis. Having lost several brothers and sisters to cancer, Dad had said many times that he hoped to die with his boots on; he did not want to die of cancer. He went into surgery hoping he would die under the knife if the polyps proved to be malignant.

They were not malignant. Dad recovered, and soon began to ponder why he had not died. He was approaching seventy-one years of age. He decided he had been given an extra year for good behavior, although he suspected that his behavior hadn't been all that good.

Less than three months after his seventy-first birthday, Dad's car hit a telephone pole on the way to his favorite clam-digging spot on the beach. He died that night during surgery. He had chosen his own time and his own way. His choice was not made at the conscious level, for his dearly loved son was with him in the car; however, he died the way he wanted to die, literally with his clam-digging boots on. (His son had minor injuries.)

o o o

From my journal:

November, 1983

"Illness," says Hutschnecker, "is an unconscious temporary surrender of the will to live." Unconscious. Temporary. And, "repeated illness is a form of slow suicide."[2] Is this recurrence "repeated illness?"

Reading Hutschnecker is frustrating, irritating, scary. If it is true, and my unconscious mind can be so destructive, doesn't that make me a helpless victim of a vicious and uncontrollable force? Am I a helpless victim of my own unconscious? That notion is more frightening than having cancer.

Though it's painful to confront this notion, in my own case it probably was true. As precious as life is, there were times in the past when it was not so precious, when circumstances seemed to conspire against me, and joy was only faintly remembered. Even now when life is filled with joy there are sometimes moments when there is a brief memory of a chill wind blowing from a black abyss, something I don't understand and only half remember. The fear of death, perhaps? The opposite of the creative force?

And what is this present joy about? How can it be that the years since I first had cancer have been filled with joy, contentment, and happiness, unlike the years before? A survivor of malignant melanoma said on a talk show recently, "The weeks after the diagnosis were the most euphoric and exhilarating of my life," a feeling I recognize. What does this mean?

o   o   o

Making death visible, bringing the fear of death to conscious awareness, and finally having all-out, open, face-to-face warfare with the Thanatos within us is revitalizing and life-giving. The Eros, the creative force, is stronger—once marshalled, the creative force enhances all aspects of life.

When one makes the decision to live, all of the energy and joy of that creative force is unleashed and life changes in a most wonderful way. As most cancer survivors will testify, once they accept the

37

challenge to fight to live, life is never again as it was before.

What do we believe about death? When I confronted my own beliefs I discovered that, to me, it was the ultimate punishment. For what? Sin, obviously. Suffering before dying was logical, as a way of prolonging the punishment. And I accepted this view because of my perception of God—as a Being separate from me, harsh and judgmental and punitive.

Our Father? Would a father punish his children for childish mistakes? And even if he would, would that punishment take the form of suffering and death? Long ago as a young mother I rejected that perception of God as a vengeful, punishing Being. How could a loving Father torment His children so? There must not be a God, I decided. I decided I was an atheist.

It has so aptly been said, "There are no atheists in the foxholes." With the second cancer came a real fear of dying, and the need to understand my relationship to "God" intensified. The word itself made me uncomfortable. As a friend pointed out, however, any belief I had in a power for good in the universe is the same as a belief in God. I resisted the word because it held connotations I could not accept.

But I could not accept a world where nothing exists beyond our limited perceptions of reality, where there is no universal creative force or power.

Nor could I accept a classical theism, a universe where God and the world are real and separate, except for some devastating or miraculous activity from God to the world.

My mother sent me a paragraph from a book called *A Course in Miracles*, published by the

Foundation for Inner Peace. It was so pointedly appropriate and comforting (though I've forgotten now what it was) that I bought my own copy of the *Course*. I read the Introduction, then I read further. In it, I recognized the truth I already knew but could not articulate. God was not as I had feared Him to be. God is within me, I am within God. Suffering and death are not punishments from God, but choices *we* make, and can unmake. God intends for us only happiness, health, peace and joy.

The *Course* describes the ego as the source of the death wish, and of the fear of God. The ego is our lower self, the part of us that believes we have separated ourselves from God—and that belief is the source of all guilt and fear. Such a belief naturally leads to an expectation of punishment: if we have separated ourselves from God, the logic goes, won't God punish us for that? And isn't death the ultimate punishment? The ego's guilt and fear expect and invite such punishment.

Our higher Self, the part of us that is in constant communication with God, knows better when we listen to it. We could not be separate from God even if we wanted to be. The separation never occurred. No guilt or punishment is necessary. Our higher Self always seeks to unify and heal.

From my journal:

January, 1984

This is tough to swallow, even though it rings true. I (or my ego) is responsible for my own illness? Worse, I chose to be sick? And even worse, was I (my ego) now choosing to die?

Why would I do that? To punish myself, perhaps, to beat God to it, to avoid eternal punishment? To stay in control, to affirm the reality of my body as having "a mind of its own?" To be a victim?

If the ego is the source of the death wish—the Thanatos—then the higher Self must be the source of the will to live, the Eros, the creative force.

I think my higher Self is what I've always felt as intuition, or conscience—the instinctive "goodness," messages from the better part of my unconscious. Apparently I've been listening to the wrong self. The lower self, which wants to die. How heartening to know that all the time, my higher Self has maintained a steady will to live, and that I can choose to tap into it at any time.

o   o   o

The fact that we are sick simply illustrates the strength and power of our mind, and of the death wish, which comes from a part of our mind. We can choose to use that strength and power to heal rather than to harm. We can choose to deny the false messages from the ego part of our mind, and to accept instead the reality of who we are, and the strength and power of our will to live.

---

[1] Hutschnecker, Arnold A., M.D., *The Will to Live*. Prentice Hall, 1951; Simon & Schuster, Cornerstone Library, 1983; p. 28

[2] Hutschnecker, *The Will to Live*, p. 34

Chapter Two

Second Stage:
Taking Charge of The Treatment

"Instead of turning fighters into victims, we should be turning victims into fighters."

Bernie Siegel, M.D.

Taking Charge of My Treatment

*W*hile still in the hospital recovering from the partial mastectomy, I saw for the first time the apparent effectiveness of positive visualization as a tool in fighting cancer. It was my first effort to participate in my treatment.

It was the third day after surgery. I still had the pathology report to get through. Was there lymph node involvement? I had done so much positive visualization it was becoming a habit, something I did every waking moment as background for whatever else was going on. It was while I was in the hospital that first time that I started to keep a journal. As my first entry, I recorded the day of the pathology report:

March 14, 1979

Today is the day the pathology lab report will come back, to tell whether or not the cancer has spread to the lymph nodes. If it has, my chances of survival drop from eighty-five percent to fifty percent or so, and I'll have to have chemotherapy. Both Dr. Fisher and Dr. Davidson insist they can feel lumps in my lymph nodes, and they are both certain it has already spread. I told Dr. Fisher that I would prove to him I could get rid of it myself, and he laughed at me. That got my anger energy going.

I've spent the week since the diagnosis doing positive visualizations night and day, as the Simontons discussed in their book. I believe I am well now, and I know those visualizations have stimulated my immune system to fight any stray cancer cells and destroy them. I feel certain of this. I haven't heard the lab report yet. But I know what it will be.

My certainty wavered this morning. Lying in bed and listening to hospital noises, fear rose like the tide. I looked for something to read to calm the panic, and there was the Gideon Bible. I remembered a trick Dad used to use, something I had smiled at for its superstition. But superstition was clearly in order now. I opened the Bible at random and without looking allowed my hand to fall on the page with the forefinger outstretched. I read the verse where my finger lay, Mark 5:34, and my mind jolted:

"And He said to her, 'Daughter, your faith has made you well; go in peace, and be healed of your affliction.'"

This verse scrambles my thoughts. It confirms what I know to be true, but can it be pure chance that this particular message comes at this particular time? It gives me comfort, and there is a part of my mind that is filled with awe in the middle of the confusion.

[Later that same day] Dr. Fisher came to see me at three o'clock, looking uncomfortable. "Well," he began, "the tests have come back." I was smiling. That made him angry. "I know what they said," I responded. He didn't like this. He is a scientist and is not superstitious. He told me he had removed eighteen nodes, and had all of them dissected. They found no sign of malignancy in any of them. He doesn't understand these results, and he appears to be angry with me for being right.

o   o   o

I had a tool to use in dealing with cancer, positive visualization and belief in my wellness. This was proof that it worked—proof enough for me.

Following surgery there was no further treatment. I saw Dr. Davidson for a checkup every three months as part of the data collection for his study. I continued to do positive affirmations and visualizations but felt no particular threat.

By Christmas I was strong enough physically and emotionally to move into an apartment and file for divorce. New Year's Day was my first day in the new apartment and the new life, and it felt wonderful. As soon as I moved out Bruce admitted that my paranoid suspicions had all been accurate, and I was utterly relieved to feel healthy and sane again. I could trust my intuition after all. I had begun to believe Bruce was right—that my mental health was failing along with my physical health.

The day after I moved out Dave told Mary to leave. After work Dave and I compared notes at a bar near the office. It was the first time we had ever discussed the affair. I asked him if he had known about it. He reflected my own feeling of relief in finally acknowledging the truth as he told me that he had known from the beginning. The difference between us was that, while he trusted his perceptions, he kept them to himself. "Why didn't you *tell* me?" I wanted to know.

"Because you weren't yet ready or able to hear it," he responded. "You had enough to deal with. I knew when you could handle it you would leave, and I just bided my time." Bided his time, and pretended nothing was wrong for six months. I had not experienced such friendship before.

The next year was one of healing. I bought a new car and a small, cozy house. I didn't feel like dating. Occasionally I had lunch with a colleague and longtime friend, Jack, a program director at the same level as I in the research organization. His wife had died two years earlier, and he was building a new life for himself, just as I was.

By the end of the year, our friendship had turned into romance, in spite of my reservations. He was a decent, loyal, honest and loving man, yet I found it hard to accept my intuition that here was someone I could always trust. By the spring of

1981, Jack had convinced me. We were married in April.

In the joy of that day and the months that followed, it seemed nothing could ever again threaten my peace of mind. We bought a farm in the Coast Range and moved there in October. We commuted to work in Portland, enjoying that daily time together. Jack's two children and my three visited often, two of them newly married themselves.

Lying in bed one night I discovered a new hardness, a growing thing in my chest beneath the flat spot where the tumor had been removed. Fear moved in and disturbed my sleep regularly. I saw the oncologist every month, asking for reassurance about the hard place, and always getting it.

From my journal:

September 26, 1982

Three years ago this month, no more cancer. I wish I were free of the fear along with the cancer. There's a hardness I've not noticed before, right below the incision. It scares me. I cancelled the Advisory Board trip to the Phoenix resort so I could see Dr. Davidson and tell him my fear. I felt guilty, because for the first time in three years I skipped my quarterly checkup September sixth. Dr. Davidson said the hard place was nothing, I was just feeling my rib. I should have gone to Phoenix.

October 28, 1982

Saw Dr. Davidson again. He still says it's nothing, but in bed I get night terrors, feeling that hard place. I can't seem to stop myself from feeling it and scaring myself. I made an appointment for December seventh, for my annual mammogram. I'm tired all the time, dragging around and forcing myself to work, but I care less and less about all the artificial deadlines and the flogging from above to produce more than is humanly possible. The constant travel and jet lag are exhausting and all the work is waiting for me when I get back to the office. Partly because I'm not sleeping well, and partly because of work pressures, I feel drained of energy and disconnected from everything—just going through the motions.

December 7, 1982

Mammogram today. I twisted around to see the bluish X-ray picture as soon as it came off the machine. There was a large area close to the breastbone that was solid light, and I panicked. A tumor! It takes days to get an interpretation of a mammogram, so I tried to call Dr. Davidson from the hospital lobby. He was out of town. I called Dr. Fisher and insisted that his nurse let me talk to him directly. I told her I had seen my mammogram and that I was certain it showed a large tumor, and I was terrified. She got him on the phone. He was his usual brusque self.

"So you're some kind of big X-ray expert now?" and, "No, I can't see you on the spur of the moment, for God's sake, come in next week. Tell the appointment desk." He was irritated that I had demanded he talk to me personally. He's retiring at the end of the month, and is really busy right now, trying to finish with all of his patients.

The appointment desk wouldn't give me an appointment until December 21. Oh well. At least it's before Christmas.

What if it's a new tumor? Will I tell anyone, before Christmas? No. If it's a tumor, I won't tell anyone yet, maybe not even Jack. All the kids will be home. It will be a special Christmas.

December 21, 1982

Dr. Fisher read my mammogram and pronounced it normal and examined me and said the hard place was my rib. He wrote it in my chart. I read it upside down while he wrote it. "Hard place is rib." And he drew a picture of where it was. It's my rib.

His retirement is only a week away, and he seemed relieved he didn't have to deal with a recurrence in a patient who has been doing so well.

I feel a little silly, and am angry that I wasted so much time and lost so much sleep worrying. What a relief. Merry Christmas!

January 20, 1983

Well, that euphoria didn't last. As soon as the Christmas furor died down, I was back to lying in bed at night feeling that growing hard place and trying not to worry. Trying not to worry keeps you awake worse than worrying. I made another appointment with Dr. Davidson. Saw him today, and told him how worried I was. This is the third time I've told him. He examined me, frowned, looked at my chart.

"What did Dr. Fisher say?" he asked.

"He says it's my rib," I told him.

He examined me again, rather carefully, and said, "Well, I think it's nothing, but let's watch it. Come back in a month."

Another month.

February 22, 1983
Laurie's twenty-first birthday

    Today I couldn't take it any longer, and I told Dr. Davidson that I knew this thing was growing; I wasn't just imagining it; I could feel it, and I just couldn't stand to keep worrying about it. What mixed feelings! I wanted to believe the doctors, hated to think about a biopsy, all the tests, surgery, and ...? I always welcomed the verdict of "It's nothing," but deep inside I never believed it. Just allowed myself to put it off for another month.

    This time Dr. Davidson agreed with me. He definitely felt something, and said it was probably a chondrosarcoma, a benign growth in the bone. He had a patient just recently with one of those. He called Dr. Michaels, a chest surgeon, and asked him to see me soon. They made an appointment for March seventh. Two more weeks. I don't believe in his "benign growth." I know what it is. I've known for six months. Everything is cold and silent and still inside me, and I feel sick, and tired.

    I have to go to New York City for the Channel 15 meeting next week. Jack will go with me, and we will stay at the Plaza Hotel, where that little girl lived. (What was her name? Eloise?) We are going to do the town. Who knows what's next? We're both scared, and neither one of us is sleeping well now.

    I'm not talking about this much with Jack. Since [his wife] Helen died of lung disease, and I seem to be having a continuing chest cancer problem, I feel sick that he might have to go through this again. No point in messing up a good trip with maudlin speculations. It might be a chondrosarcoma.

March 7, 1983

Dr. Michaels said it's a large tumor, and scheduled surgery for next Monday, March 11. Three and a half years to the day after my first surgery. I will go to the annual Planning Retreat tomorrow, but I'll have to tell them that I'll be taking a six-week leave. I feel numb. And reluctant to tell people about this. I wonder what that's about? It's just that it's so personal, something I should keep private.

March 9, 1983

People at work are stunned, quiet, and supportive. Dave's first wife had cancer recurrences several times. Then she died. He doesn't expect me to live, I can tell. But I will.

o   o   o

While Jack and I waited in pre-op my brother Tim found us and settled in for the day, playing hookey from his teaching job to give us both jokes and tough love, and to buy Jack drinks with lunch while they waited. My mother arrived as I was wheeled off the elevator on the way to surgery, and the little girl in me who wanted to crawl up in her lap settled for a quick, grateful hug.

I woke on the way out of surgery, on a gurney headed for the recovery room. Dr. Michaels was walking beside me, leaning over the gurney, and he said, "It was a recurrence of your breast cancer, and you will need to have chemotherapy."

I knew what that meant: the prognosis was bleak. I went right back to sleep, grateful for the blessing of anesthesia.

For two days I drifted in and out of a peaceful sleep, waking long enough to register that Jack was sitting by my bed, holding my hand, watching me with focused intensity, willing me to be well. His quiet presence was immensely comforting, and I floated in an insulating cocoon of love for those two days of blessed intermission.

Soon enough, I had to wake up.

This tumor was a recurrence beneath the chest wall, the size of an orange—why did they always use food analogies? According to my doctors the new growth was obviously a metastasis. This meant the cancer had begun from cells transmitted through the blood or lymph system rather than growing from local cells left behind from the first tumor. Dr. Michaels, was cheerfully emphatic. I would need radiation and chemotherapy. But of course Dr. Davidson, would need to concur with his opinion.

Dr. Michaels sent me across town to another hospital for six weeks of radiation treatments. I met radiation oncologist Dr. Roberts who would become one of my favorites—he was brash, irreverent, and obviously bright and well informed. After examining me his first question was, "Since you only had a lumpectomy, why didn't you have radiation therapy as followup?"

"I didn't know it was an option," I replied, astonished at his question. "I was told that no one knew if radiation was appropriate as a followup treatment, and that I didn't need it."

Dr. Roberts assured me that had I come to his hospital I might still have had a lumpectomy, but would most certainly have followed that surgery with radiation therapy, since in 1979 it was the treatment of choice, following lumpectomy.

I quizzed him exhaustively, shocked that there had been an option I had not been told about. Still, had I asked? Not really. I had asked few questions then, and had accepted without question the recommended course of treatment.

In 1979 few surgeons were willing to experiment with this less radical surgery. Those who did usually chose the conservative option of followup radiation therapy to the affected area of the breast. In my case, though, I had agreed to be part of a research study designed to find out for certain if the conservative option was in fact necessary.

The five-year results of that study are now in, and it is clear that simple lumpectomy must be followed by radiation therapy to be as effective as a complete mastectomy.

I was angry. I felt not just misled, but lied to. Had Dr. Davidson been so eager to secure subjects for his study that he had not fully informed mé of the treatment options? I stormed over to his office and asked to see his research assistant, who had explained the consent form to me more than three years earlier. After telling her of the fix I was in now I demanded to know why I had not been fully informed. I insisted on seeing the consent form I had signed, which didn't discuss radiation at all.

I was out of control. The research assistant was pale and trembling, unable to respond to my questions. This was the nightmare any clinical researcher fears: a patient in the "no treatment" group who, it turns out, should have received treatment. She was unprepared to handle it.

The research assistant left the office and returned a few minutes later, telling me, "Dr. Davidson wants to see you right away." This was the fastest I had ever gotten in to see a doctor.

I had begun to take charge of my treatment.

o   o   o

Dr. Davidson was agitated and defensive. We had a heated, difficult discussion, and I asked him to tell me what the prognosis was, now that I had had a major recurrence. He was blunt, not inclined toward gentleness with this pugnacious, enraged woman in his face. "Only five percent of women who have had chest wall metastases survived for three years after the recurrence. There's a ninety-five percent chance that you'll have another metastasis soon."

"How soon?" I asked.

"Within three months, I'd guess," he replied.

"And what are my chances of survival after that?"

"Zero."

I was still too angry to be horrified at this prognosis. I challenged his figures, no longer trusting anything he told me. I demanded to know the source of these statistics. There were three studies, he told me, and only three, that had been done on women with chest wall recurrences of breast cancer. Only five percent had survived three years, even with radiation and chemotherapy. In most cases, further recurrences had followed in quick succession.

I asked about radiation and chemotherapy for me. It was his judgment that radiation therapy was indeed called for now, but not chemotherapy. He saw no point in using debilitating drugs when the prognosis was so negative.

During my next appointment with Dr. Michaels I asked him again about the chemotherapy he had repeatedly recommended. This time he wasn't so sure. He thought probably I didn't need chemotherapy after all.

"Have you been talking to Dr. Davidson?" I asked him.

He smiled, wryly. He had been talking to Dr. Davidson. His nonverbal language said it all. One does have the right to disagree with authority in the privacy of one's own convictions—"Sir Thomas" was the affectionate but semi-serious way he referred to Dr. Davidson today.

I decided it was time for a second opinion, and probably time to consider changing oncologists.

With the first tumor it seemed there had been no decisions to make. I simply accepted the recommendations of my doctors without question. Now I realized that if I had pursued even one second opinion I would no doubt have learned of the experimental nature of the treatment being recommended to me. It might have been confusing to learn of the range of treatment options that existed. I might have made the same choice even knowing the options. But had it been truly my informed choice I would have been more willing to take responsibility for the outcomes of those decisions.

I chose to remain ignorant that first time, allowing the doctors to preempt my own decision-making responsibilities.

This time was different. By now it was clear to me that there was no single, clear-cut indisputable answer, and that even the doctors disagreed about the best course to follow. I bought a book by Rose Kushner, *Why Me?*, which exhaustively reviewed all of the breast cancer treatment alternatives. She discussed the long-term study I had been a part of.

Of the experimental "no treatment" group that I was in, she writes:

"This group of women is being treated only by segmental surgery [a lumpectomy] and an axillary dissection [underarm lymph node removal]: no radiotherapy is being given at all. At this time, survival rates are equal enough to allow the study to continue. If, after ten, fifteen, or twenty years, there is no difference between survival rates of these women and of those whose breasts were irradiated, this will be proof that the X-ray treatments were not needed. The results won't be in until the end of the clinical trials, however, so *most breast-cancer experts believe everything possible must be done to try to destroy any hidden centricles in the rest of the breast* [by radiotherapy]." (Emphasis mine.)

This sounded like information that, in the interests of medical ethics, should have been given to me before I was asked to sign a consent form and become part of a research study.

The rest of the book told me more than I really wanted to know about chemotherapy.

Armed with this information I made an appointment to see Dr. Boles, the oncologist said to be the most aggressive in treating cancer. He examined me carefully, reviewed my case, and spent an hour talking with Jack and me about the options and the prognosis.

Dr. Boles recommended that radiation therapy be followed by chemotherapy, and he would use a combination of three drugs: 5-FU (Fluorourocyl),

Methotrexate, and Adriamycin, all highly toxic. But from Kushner's book I knew that Adriamycin could also affect the heart. I asked why he chose Adria-mycin. His response was that it was the most aggressive drug against advanced breast cancers, and he saw no point in using something less powerful and taking the chance that it wouldn't stop the progress of the cancer.

"Is mine an advanced breast cancer?" I asked Dr. Boles. "Couldn't it simply be a one-time local recurrence?"

No, he didn't think so. The new tumor had developed on the inside of the chest wall. Cancer cells couldn't have passed through the chest wall, he told us. This had to have been a metastasis—a spread to a distant organ, in this case the inside of the chest wall—by traveling via the bloodstream or lymphatic system. That meant I was very likely to have further metastases.

Dr. Boles quoted the same three studies, and again, ninety-five percent chance of further recurrences. In his opinion, there was only one possible course of action: immediate, aggressive chemotherapy, begun as soon as radiation therapy was completed. I questioned him further about the three studies, and he offered to make copies of them for me to read. I accepted, gratefully.

As a trained researcher myself, I found major flaws in the studies. They were based on historical data, that is, information gathered after the fact about women who could be located and for whom medical records were available. Women who had chest wall recurrences and got well were not likely to check back in for the sake of research. I was not willing to base my own probability of getting well on only three studies of such dubious certainty. The way I saw it, my chances were either 100 percent or zero, and no one could predict what my specific, unique probability would be.

Dr. Roberts, the radiation oncologist, also believed chemotherapy was called for. I asked him to recommend someone for a third opinion. I wasn't sure it was necessary to use Adriamycin except as a last resort. I just didn't feel, at this point, that things were that desperate. I would rather save Adriamycin for later, in case the more traditional chemotherapy didn't work. If I took it now there would be no backup if one were needed.

Dr. Paul was my third opinion. He knew of the three studies—in fact, had trained at M.D. Anderson Hospital in Houston where the studies were carried out. Nevertheless, he wasn't willing to talk about statistics or probabilities. He apparently recognized the danger in using group statistics to make predictions about individuals. The chemotherapy he recommended was a conservative combination of 5-FU, Methotrexate, and Cytoxan. Cytoxan, while still highly toxic, was not known to cause heart damage. I liked this option better—I intended to survive this with my heart intact.

I changed to a new medical insurance plan during an open enrollment period at work, and chose Dr. Paul as my new oncologist. He was young, gently courteous and oddly formal, not a man I could warm up to quickly. But he appeared to be knowledgeable and competent and was willing to let me believe I could get well. I knew the importance of a good relationship with one's doctor, and doubted that Dr. Paul and I would ever be on a first-name basis, but he felt right to me. He was the only doctor I'd seen yet who would try to transcend the tyranny of statistics.

I was beginning to feel more in control of what was happening to me. I did have decisions to make and with Jack's support I was making them. Some of our discussions were difficult—it's hard to talk about "saving Adriamycin as a last resort in case the first chemo doesn't work." We were both in denial, both certain of a positive outcome whatever the treatment. We saw the doctors, medicines and treatments as agents giving tangible form to my choice—my choice to be healed.

All necessary decisions had now been made. Radiation therapy had begun two weeks after surgery, and chemotherapy would begin two weeks after radiation ended.

Life returned to normal—as normal as it ever could be in my experience. I accepted a teaching job at the university, resigned my other job, and took the summer off to recuperate. We were in the throes of remodeling. Jack refused to "carry Sheetrock up and down the stairs at my age." A crew of from two to six carpenters tramped through steadily all summer long, working on the upstairs which we were turning into guest rooms and a dormitory.

Mike graduated from college and in July my first grandson was born. Being present at the birth was an indescribably joyful experience. Jordan was born at four o'clock in the morning, allowing me to feel the full impact of going without sleep while in chemo.

Within two weeks the new family moved in with us at the farm until Mike could find a job. He was discouraged with the realities of the job market. An honors degree in physics was not enough to give automatic, immediate entry into the high tech jobs he sought. In three months the right opportunity came along and they moved to Portland.

Those three months were in many ways life-giving to me. The presence of the new baby gave me constant assurance of the durability of the life force and the innocence and sweetness of human beings. A gratifying bonding process was taking place with this tiny grandson. My children were there with love and support for me during a difficult time. The unfinished attic, former home to spiders, bats and mice, was turning into a comfortable refuge. In September I started the new job teaching at the university and wore a wig to classes to cover my patchy baldness.

It was clear that life was not going to hold still while I worked out the details of having cancer.

The Need to Feel in Control

The patient's job in managing her treatment has several facets. First she must be in charge of the medical aspects of her recovery. Her doctor is an important expert resource. He or she has the knowledge, training, skills and experience to recommend the best medical options and to help the patient get the most worthwhile treatment. Her doctor will monitor the effectiveness of the treatment, make constant adjustments, and help her find ways to avoid side effects. Doctor and patient can be a team, and the patient plays at least as important a role on that team as does her doctor.

At the same time, perhaps the patient's most important task is to nourish and support her own immune system, which is her first line of defense. This is particularly true if she is receiving radiotherapy or chemotherapy—both are immunosuppressive. So is surgery or any other assault on the body, mind, or emotions. But the good news is that boosting her immune system is something she can do for herself, and it's free. There is little that the medical establishment can do, yet, to reinforce one's immune responses (although promising research is being done), but there is a great deal that the patient can do.

In the next chapter I will describe several of the ways patients can strengthen their immune systems. But first, they will need to get their treatment under way and under control.

We all have a need to feel in charge of our lives. We feel particularly vulnerable at times when events seem to be beyond our ability to affect the outcome. Cancer is one of those times. And yet, it's an important time to feel in control—necessary to our recovery.

The immune system is our most powerful defense against cancer, and not feeling in control has a negative effect on its function. One interesting experiment by psychologist Mark Laudenslager at the University of Denver demonstrated the effect of helplessness on the immune system. Laudenslager and his colleagues gave mild electric shocks to twenty-four rats. Half the rats could turn off the current by turning a wheel in their cage, and the other half could not. The rats in the two groups were paired so that each time a rat turned the wheel its helpless partner also was protected from the shock.

The researchers found that the helpless rats, who could not *choose* to turn the wheel, showed an immune system response depressed below normal. The rats who were in charge responded normally. Both groups of rats had a remedy for the shock, but only one was in control of the remedy. What the researchers had demonstrated, they believe, was that lack of control over an event, not the experience itself, is what weakens the immune system.[3]

Psychiatrists believe from similar experiments with rats and from observations of human subjects that being helpless, or feeling helpless, is one of the most harmful factors in depression.

It's difficult to feel in control during a conversation with one's doctor. He (or she) is usually standing, dressed in all the symbols of authority: white coat, stethoscope and blooming good health. You, on the other hand, are sitting on the edge of a table with your bare feet dangling, dressed in a baby blue garment which barely covers your fanny. You are scared; your doctor is in a hurry.

It's difficult to feel in control when weakened by illness, surgery, radiation, chemotherapy, or other debilitating treatments. Or when your hair has fallen out.

The body you once trusted to be strong and well has betrayed you.

It doesn't help that some of your acquaintances let you know by their words or actions that they expect you to die. In my case, one well-meaning acquaintance let me know her expectation in a little speech thanking me for the professional help I had given her. We had never before had such a conversation and there was no small talk around her expression of gratitude. We met at a conference cocktail party, she said what she had to say and moved on as if a duty had been discharged while there was still time. She has not communicated with me in the years since. While I appreciated the kind words, the unspoken message was clear: I don't expect ever to see you again.

In the face of these threats to your control over what happens to you, you can and should find ways to take charge, to feel that you are not helpless, not a victim but a competent person, managing events even when they seem out of control.

The patient risks antagonizing her doctor when she insists on being in charge of what happens to her. Some doctors don't appreciate an amateur (the patient) meddling in what they consider to be exclusively their domain. Bernie Siegel suggests in his book that if you have this type of doctor you should immediately change doctors. On the other hand, depending on your personality, you may welcome the sparring match and may find it a pleasure to teach your doctor a thing or two about patients.

Several research studies with breast cancer patients have shown that those patients judged by their doctors to be most difficult and demanding— asked the most questions and expressed their emotions freely—had the best likelihood of long-term survival. Leonard Derogatis, a psychologist, found that long-term survivors had poor relationships with their physicians (according to the physicians).[4]

Sandra Levy found that seriously ill breast-cancer patients who expressed their emotions such as depression, anxiety and hostility, survived longer than those who showed little distress. Psychologist Levy and others have shown that aggressive, difficult patients tend to have more killer T cells (the immune system "seek and destroy" cells) than do docile, uncomplaining patients.[5]

A group of researchers in London reported the results of a long-term study showing that cancer patients who reacted to the diagnosis with a fighting spirit had a ten-year survival rate of seventy-five percent, compared with a twenty-two percent survival rate for those who responded with stoic acceptance or feelings of helplessness or hopelessness.[6]

I felt vindicated by these studies. I knew that I had become an increasingly difficult patient, no longer willing to simply accept whatever doctors recommended to me. According to this research my attitude probably helped to save my life.

Acceptance comes later. For now you need accept nothing unless you choose to. And don't doubt for a moment that your doctors are familiar with the research I have just cited—they know their most difficult patients are also the ones who are most likely to survive, and survival is a feather in their cap as well as yours.

Dealing With Doctors

I now had three doctors: Dr. Michaels, who continued with surgical followup; Dr. Roberts, radiation oncologist; and Dr. Paul, my new primary physician and oncologist. Dr. Paul specialized in hematology, particularly the changes in blood caused by some cancers and by chemotherapy treatment. I liked and trusted them all but was from time to time furious with one or another of them, in out-and-out disagreement on basic principles. Each relationship varied at times from mutual respect to mutual frustration.

I asked Dr. Roberts if he knew Dr. Simonton, the author of *Getting Well Again*. They were both radiation oncologists, after all. It turned out they had gone to medical school together, and Dr. Roberts was not pleased to admit it. He considered the techniques the Simontons were using to be "quackery, as silly as coffee enemas." The remarkable results the Simontons achieved with their techniques could not to be given credence—they were depending on the power of the patient's own mind and spirit.

"But they use those techniques as a *supplement* to medical therapy, not as a substitute," I protested.

It made no difference. Someone might get the idea she could forgo traditional treatment in favor of meditative fantasies, for heaven's sake. Dr. Roberts apparently could not have an open mind about this. I was surprised—in every other way he was most progressive, informed, and humane, often appearing on television to talk about the most recent techniques in breast cancer treatment. Come to think of it, he didn't discuss visualization as one of those techniques.

My original oncologist, Dr. Davidson, had reacted similarly to my questions about positive visualization in treating cancer. Yet years later I heard that he was himself involved in a research project with Dr. Simonton. Perhaps my question about it, and the questions of many other patients, led him to give the issue a second look.

When I asked questions about nutrition Dr. Paul was vague and uninformed. That wasn't his field. When I told him I was using mental and spiritual techniques to supplement chemo, his cheery reply was, "Well, it certainly can't do any harm." As long as I took his medicine, I could do whatever else I liked with no argument from him.

In seeking out additional medical opinions, I learned some important and surprising things about doctors:

- ••• Doctors sometimes are wrong (probably at least as often as I am, which is a lot),
- ••• Doctors sometimes make mistakes (at least as often as I do...),
- ••• Doctors often disagree with each others' medical opinions, techniques, or philosophies,
- ••• Doctors sometimes change their minds,
- ••• Doctors sometimes are afraid of cancer, and
- ••• doctors can, and often do, learn from their patients.

Further, although doctors are exhaustively trained in their specialties they receive little training which might prepare them to deal with the emotional, mental, and spiritual aspects of disease. They deal with statistical generalities and apply them to individual cases, because that is the scientific way. As non-scientists, we reason the other way around—our own case is primary to us, so our only reality is our personal experience. Both are valid and necessary ways of thinking, and both should be valued.

In dealing with doctors we need to be ready to point out that any time a miracle occurs, such as a permanent remission of cancer when one seemed impossible, it is important evidence. If it can happen for one person, it can happen for anyone. Those of us who are not wearing the blinders of scientific objectivity (not to be confused with scientific curiosity) have seen and heard of enough miracles to convince ourselves without a doubt that they happen routinely.

When I decided to take charge of my own treatment, I considered the following: I bring to the decision-making process a wealth of information that the doctors cannot have. I have lived with my body all my life. Even though in 1979 I was unaccustomed to paying attention to and listening to my body, I gradually learned to note the subtle changes, the intuition that something is wrong, even before I had the visible symptoms. I learned to trust that I knew when I was getting better, even before the doctors did. I knew when a medicine was doing more harm than good. I got used to paying attention to myself and I see myself daily. The doctor sees me less frequently, and understandably has a hard time remembering the small but so-important details.

What better person to place in charge of your treatment than yourself? Who knows you better? Who has a greater interest in a successful outcome? And who never, ever, keeps you waiting for hours with nothing to read but *People* magazine?

Now that you're in charge, you're going to be busy. Even though you may have already made some decisions or accepted some recommendations without question, it is never too late to reconsider. You should feel free to change doctors if you find you have made an unfortunate choice. The supply of physicians has begun to exceed the demand in many cities, and you may find yourself in an excellent position to shop around.

First, no matter how much you trust your doctor, get a second opinion. Get a second perspective, a totally different combination of experience and training and belief. Then remember it's called a second opinion because that's just what it is— somebody's opinion.

Human beings are so variable and unpredictable that no doctor can say for certain, ever, what the verdict is for you as a specific human being. There is *no* kind of disease that has not been cured, including AIDS. Doctors can tell you the diagnosis, and you can and should accept that. But you don't have to accept the prognosis, so get a second opinion. If the two opinions differ greatly, get a third. No single doctor has a cornerstone on wisdom or insight. It is your wisdom and your insight that will have to put it all together.

If you have just received a diagnosis you may feel that you don't have time to seek other opinions, to get the information and to do the thinking. You may believe that the situation is urgent and that you must make a decision fast. Seldom is it truly urgent that treatment decisions be made immediately. A few days to give careful consideration to all the options probably will not affect the outcome. On the other hand, your feeling that you are in control of what happens to you *can* affect the outcome, for the better.

Next, while you are seeking out medical opinion, you will be in a better position to evaluate the options and to stay in charge if you inform yourself. There is a variety of resources available to you as you seek information. Your nearest chapter of the American Cancer Society (ACS) can answer questions and can provide a number of helpful booklets. The National Cancer Institute, a division of the National Institutes of Health, also provides booklets, and some of the diet and nutrition booklets are particularly helpful.

The ACS or your doctor can give you a list of support groups of cancer patients and their families who meet regularly to provide information and mutual support and encouragement. Many hospitals have counseling available for cancer patients and their families, and your doctor or nurse should be able to help you find out about such services.

You may be, as I am, a reader. I found a section of cancer books at the county library and read my way through it. If you need more information than you can get from your doctor, start reading. A list of some of the books I read, with my comments, can be found at the end of this book. My favorites are starred (*) and can be used to lay a foundation for the work of getting well. New books on the subject are published every day. I often scour the largest bookstores for new titles, then go to the library and request that the books be ordered.

Finally, when you have sought several different medical opinions and have informed yourself, you are ready to select a doctor.

Friends who have had cancer have told me of their wonderful, nurturing, positive, loving, hope-giving, supportive doctors. Although my doctors were certainly competent and kind I never met such a paragon in my own encounters, and I wondered why. Some of my doctors brushed off or laughed at my own attempts to use metaphysical and spiritual strategies. Most patronized me in my belief system. One told me that writing this book would probably be therapeutic for me, even though it wouldn't be published. Why was I finding doctors who were so opposed to all that I found helpful?

It wasn't until recently that I realized these doctors were the best I could have found, given my personality. Since childhood, when I have encountered disbelief in my abilities, from friends or supervisors, I responded with angry determination to "show them." When told that something couldn't be done, I mulishly resolved to prove that I could do it. Anger mobilized my energies, and fueled my own healing work. When Dr. Davidson told me I would have another recurrence within three months, and after that a zero chance of survival, I promised myself that I would outlive him. That angry determination may have helped me to get well more than any amount of tender, compassionate understanding from a doctor could have.

Years after my silent vow to outlive him I nearly bumped into Dr. Davidson entering an elevator as I was leaving it. I couldn't resist glancing back. He was frozen, holding the elevator open and staring after me in open-mouthed disbelief. It was an intoxicating moment.

My own personality, then, determined how I selected a doctor, and my psychology apparently dictated that I choose the seeming opposite of the type I thought I wanted. No helpful, loving, positive supporters for me—I relished the challenge of a doctor who didn't necessarily share my beliefs.

Consider your own personality. Do you tend to internalize and accept negative predictions made about you? Do you especially believe the words of authority figures such as teachers, doctors and politicians? If that is true about you, you should look for a doctor who will help you maintain your faith in your own ability to heal. Look for a doctor who is eager to evoke and capitalize upon your own will to live, even if it means both of you must ignore or defy the probabilities. Look for positive, nurturing doctors who believe in you.

Dealing With Your Doctor

Interacting with your doctor after you have selected one can sometimes be complicated. You will have frequent questions. The danger in asking them all is that your doctor will, like mine, feel compelled to answer them in more detail than you are willing to hear, throwing in a few gloomy predictions for good measure. If you have doctors like this, you may have to be ready to stop them if what they are saying starts to scare you.

I admire a friend in chemotherapy who, when her doctor told her, "Your whole system could shut down at any time," held up her hand and told him, "Stop! I'm not going to let you scare me to death again. I intend to get well whether you believe it or not, and my system is going to continue to function just fine." He accepted her declaration with grace and good humor. She got well.

You may have to ask your doctor to help you by using, or not using, particular terminology. The powerful effect of words on our mental and emotional state cannot be overstated.

In my case, I asked my doctors not to use the words "in remission."

Well-meaning people who hear that I have completed treatment and now have no sign of cancer often ask, "How long have you been in remission?" I gently correct them. "I am not in remission. I am well. I have been well for several years, and have no reason to believe I will not stay well." To me, the word remission holds a guarantee that the cancer will eventually return. Why not decide instead that a person who has no sign of cancer is cured? If it turns out later that you were wrong and the cancer returns, what has been lost?

"In the presence of uncertainty," the Simontons point out, "there is nothing wrong with hope."

Blessings on the doctor who examines you and then asks you to get dressed and come to his or her office to discuss your case. This places you in a position to feel somewhat more in charge of yourself and your responses, and you are more likely to be able to listen carefully and to understand and process what the doctor is telling you. You are not in a position of semi-naked vulnerability and will be more able to treat the doctor as a peer and colleague, co-healer with you. If your doctor chooses to discuss your case and your options as you sit on the edge of the examining table, ask that you be allowed to get dressed and sit in a chair before continuing the discussion. You may also ask that your spouse, son or daughter, friend or parent in the waiting room be allowed to join you for the discussion.

It was my experience that when the topic was very serious in its implications for me, Jack often was better able than I to listen with objectivity and to ask pertinent questions. It could not have been easy for him, either, but four ears hear better than two, and two minds remember better than one. Afterward I could review and discuss the entire conversation with Jack, and reinforce my understanding of what was said and what was meant.

While too much information and statistics can overwhelm and frighten you, you may be, as I was, the kind of person who feels better having a lot of information about what is happening. If you have this need to know and understand what can be expected, it is your right to be told anything about your disease or your treatment that you want to know. It is your absolute right to ask your doctor as many questions as you have, and it is his responsibility to answer them. If your doctor is too busy to give a satisfactory answer, ask the nurse. If the nurse can't answer, go to the American Cancer Society. If they can't answer, join one of the groups they recommend, and keep asking until you get an answer.

It is important to remember, however, that answers from medical sources are not infallible—they are simply more data to consider along with your own experience, knowledge and intuition. Many of the answers are based on studies which are used to make probability statements about your unique situation, which in my view is never appropriate. Even if a certain outcome was observed in 100 percent of the cases studied, the possibility of a different outcome in your specific case is always possible—particularly if you reject the negative prognosis for yourself.

When I had questions to ask my doctor I was easily intimidated by his aura of extreme busyness, and by the number of people still lined up in the waiting room. If he was terse or seemed irritated, I would forget most of my questions, or forget to follow up on his answers. It helped to write down the questions in advance, and even to rehearse them. And I found that he was more likely to take the time to listen and to respond if I warned him, "I have a list of questions for you," before I pulled out my list. It also helped to call ahead and ask the nurse to set aside fifteen extra minutes for questions, or thirty minutes if the list was long.

If you make such a list don't edit it as you ask the questions. No question is silly or trivial if it is of concern to you. You have a right to ask and you have a right to expect a thoughtful answer. It is important to your feeling of being in control, not helpless, that you can get information when you need it. If you are worried about side effects or symptoms, ask. You are the only person in the world who knows what you are experiencing, and no one will be able to help you unless you ask for help.

I made occasional use of the university medical school, calling a specialist to ask questions. My foot in the door was a nurse at the medical school, a friend of a friend. I called the nurse first and asked her which doctor or doctors I might be able to call with a short question. She gave me several names and numbers with their permission, and when I called them I always mentioned that I had been referred by her. After I discovered the value of a second opinion I also felt free to buy time from another doctor if I had questions my own doctor couldn't or wouldn't answer.

Just call and make an appointment, being sure to say that you will need half an hour or more, and that it is for a second opinion. It may cost several hundred dollars for an hour of a specialist's time, but it may be worth it to you to have that undivided attention and specialized expertise. Many health insurance companies will pay for a second opinion.

When you get your answer remember that what you have is one person's opinion. Granted, it is based on experience, training, and statistics from research studies, but that person doesn't know *you* and is not infallible. There is no single answer to cancer, and there is no agreement among doctors as to the single best way to treat any particular kind of cancer.

One question I learned never to ask is this one: *"Doctor, what are my chances?"*

It is a silly question, because no human being can tell you. Your chances are either 100 percent or zero percent. *You* have a lot to do with determining what your chances are, and predictions based on statistical probability may be interesting, but have nothing to do with you.

If you hear (as I did) that you have a five percent or less chance of survival, decide that you'll be in the five percent. Maybe the other ninety-five percent didn't know about their ability to affect the outcome of their disease. Maybe they wanted to die. Maybe the studies which produced the statistics were flawed. Maybe a lot of things. In any case those are numbers that are absolutely meaningless in terms of your probability of recovery. Your unique probability of survival cannot be determined by any study, by any doctor, by any set of statistics.

Establishing Your Expectations of Success

When you have completed your information gathering and processing and made all treatment decisions, the time has come to stop asking questions unless you experience problems with the treatment. This is the time when your own mental and spiritual work and your own expectations of success become paramount. You need not disturb that healing pattern by continually injecting worrisome negative predictions.

A year into chemotherapy, during one of my physical exams, I asked Dr. Paul a question. I was doing well, had no sign of cancer, and felt absolutely positive about my ultimate victory. It seemed a simple question to me, but I wrote it down and rehearsed it before asking: "What effect will long-term chemotherapy have on my immune system?"

From my reading I knew that we all have cancer cells, which the immune system constantly attacks and destroys—unless the immune system is weakened by stress, conflict, grief, pain or illness. Or chemotherapy drugs? If chemotherapy doctors hadn't yet learned how to protect the good cells while destroying the bad ones, then what would become of my immune system's advance guard, the attack cells?

Sitting on the edge of the examination table in the short gown, with Dr. Paul standing near the door in his white coat and stethoscope, I asked the question, rehearsal-perfect,

"What effect will long-term chemotherapy have on my immune system?"

In retrospect, I can see that asking the question triggered Dr. Paul's conviction that chemotherapy was my only faint hope, and his fear that I might elect to stop treatment. It was all he had to offer me, and I was questioning it.

"You have to understand," he lectured me, "you are in a perilous position. With chemotherapy we hope to keep you going, and the effect on your immune system must be seen as insignificant in relation to that."

I parried: "But the three studies showed that five percent of the women in my position survived. I intend to be in that five percent."

He counterattacked: "But one must assume that those women had tiny relapses, and you have had a quite nasty one."

I don't remember the rest of the conversation except that it ended soon. Other patients were waiting. I left the office and started the long drive home to the farm in shock and panic. Yes, I had heard it all before, and yes, this still sounded a lot like "Zero." But by now I was in charge of my own recovery, and expected to stay well and live long. This was a blow of the wrecker's ball to the carefully constructed fortress of my expectations.

On the drive home I didn't see the new spring greens, the valleys filled with low mists, the color of the sky. I planned my funeral. I reviewed my will. I raged at God, then apologized and made promises. I cried. I rehearsed deathbed scenes and wrote mental letters to my children. Cancelled plans for the summer. Made up some more deals God might find appealing. Considered driving over the cliff at the bad curve at the top of the pass. Then gradually stopped crying and cursing and started to reclaim the peace that lately had prevailed inside.

I walked into the kitchen, being strong and brave. Jack was waiting. "How did the treatment go?" he asked. I couldn't speak.

When the story had been told and I had regained some composure, my husband made a quiet observation. "A few hours ago you were a strong, confident, healthy human being. Now suddenly you are dying. What happened? The doctor said a few *words*, that's all."

Jack gave me some different words, reminding me of the path I was on, the structure I had built, my own deep inner conviction, and his, that I was now finished with illness. We retraced our steps to my present wellness, my struggle to get there, my refusal to accept the dire speculations of the medical community, my own plan for getting well and staying well.

The illusion was denied, and the illusion faded. Reality reasserted itself. I was the expert on my own wellness, not the doctor. I spent twenty-four hours a day knowing how well I was, and he still had to read my chart every time I came in for treatment, to remember the facts of my case. My own plan, my own understanding of my condition were not in the chart. And now it was time for dinner.

The next morning I woke with renewed joy and energy. Clearly, I was well. Jack made me promise not to ask Dr. Paul any more questions. We were not going to jeopardize our own system, which was working, by hearing more negative predictions. Dr. Paul would realize in time that it was useless to make predictions about me. The time to ask questions was past. We had gathered all the information there was to gather, and processed all of it. All that was to be done now was to get well.

Being in charge of my treatment, I was learning, was to invite the determined efforts of the medical community to stay in control of what they knew best. I had to let Dr. Paul know how I felt. I was still intimidated somewhat by his distance, his jammed schedule and his beliefs. So I wrote a note to give him before my next treatment. I found a card with a picture of a small, frightened mouse cowering beneath an elephant's huge upraised foot.

I composed this message for the card:

"This is how I went home feeling after all those statistical predictions. But then I remembered the Outlyer Mouse. When I was in graduate school a fellow student told me about an experiment he was involved in: mice were injected with a tranquilizer and dropped into a tank of water. Students recorded how long each mouse would swim before it sank and had to be rescued. The data produced a lovely, symmetrical, bell-shaped curve, the predictable 'normal' curve.

Until the Outlyer Mouse.

She was dropped into the tank and she swam, and swam and swam. The students watched, aghast, as their lovely 'normal' curve was skewed and more skewed by her unpredictable behavior. Finally in frustration one student reached into the tank, pushed the mouse to the bottom and held her down. Her data was thrown out and the curve returned to normal.

The moral of this allegory is: I chose you as my doctor because you told me, 'Each patient is an individual and statistics don't necessarily apply to that individual.' That perspective is important to me. When you look at me, think of the mouse swimming with great enjoyment and durability. I am an Outlyer Mouse, and together we are going to keep me swimming."

Dr. Paul read the card without comment and never again made scary predictions. Nor did I tempt him by asking loaded questions.

Nothing has ever made me feel so hemmed in, restricted and controlled as being in treatment. Daily trips to the basement radiology lab every weekday for six weeks, rain or shine, feeling well or unwell, willing or unwilling—I went. Tattooed and trussed, laid on a slab and wheeled under the ominous machine, watching as everyone in attendance took cover behind thick lead walls, it was hard to believe that this treatment was going to be good for me.

Then the chemotherapy. Months, years of presenting myself on time for the needle, trying not to remember that the stuff in the bottles was poison. Feeling liberated after the last treatment in each five-week cycle, hoping maybe my blood count would drop so low they would have to wait an exra week before beginning the next cycle. Feeling it would never end, that I'd spend my life tethered to the I.V. bottle. Minding it more than I had thought I would when my hair thinned to frail straw and came out in patches, leaving me looking like a middle-aged punk rocker.

I very much needed to find a way to feel in control while in treatment.

I found myself at times more afraid of the effects of the treatment than I was of the cancer. If the radiant rays and toxic drugs were strong enough to kill cancer cells, what were they doing to the rest of my cells, the healthy ones? The answer was clear. Any cell in the process of dividing, as cancer cells usually are, was zapped. That meant cells lining the stomach (hence, nausea), hair cells, and blood cells. The number of white cells dropped dramatically after treatment—so did the red cell and platelet count.

I knew from *Getting Well Again* what imagery, affirmation and visualization could do. These techniques had not cured me, and I no longer wanted to trust that they would, but I was willing to use them in dealing with the effects of treatment.

Cancer cells are not strong and powerful but weak and sleazy. They die easily. I visualized any cancer cells in my body as resembling cooked oatmeal, gray and soft and mushy, no match for radiation or drugs. Radiation I visualized as laser-like rays vaporizing the oatmeal, while chemotherapy drugs dissolved it.

I still worried about what all this treatment was doing to my healthy cells. Would it destroy my immune system...since the immune system is made up of blood cells? I needed to be strong to fight the cancer. I needed all my healthy cells. And I felt that lying under the linear accelerator absorbing rays while feeling worried and panicky could not provide the best environment for radiation to do its work.

I invented a regimen for myself to cope with radiation. I tried to meditate or talk myself into a calm frame of mind before going in. Often it helped to talk to others in the waiting room and reassure them or joke with them. Then while the attendants put me on the table, positioned the equipment over me and left the room, I used those few minutes to close my eyes and do my visualization.

First I talked to my healthy cells, telling them to relax, to slow down, to stop dividing. I told them to take a nap. Then I imagined light (I chose green, but one could pick any color that communicates healing) pouring in through the top of my head and washing down through my body, filling my chest cavity with green, glowing, healing, protective light. I imagined the healthy cells becoming invisible in the light, and the cancer cells standing out for the rays to find. I kept this image in my mind until the treatment was over.

I used a different strategy for chemotherapy. Since each treatment took about an hour I seldom was able to keep a visualization going for the whole time. Instead I tried again to meditate or consciously relax in the waiting room. When the I.V. was started I again mentally talked to my healthy cells, telling them to lie low for a while. Knowing the biofeedback research on how human beings can actually slow their heartbeats, raise or lower their body temperatures, or *alter cell activity* purely with the power of their thoughts, this was no idle exercise. I talked to the cancer cells, too. I told them, "Dance, suckers!"

I have no way to prove that these strategies actually had an effect on my response to treatment. I do know, however, that my method was far preferable to the fear, panic, resistance, and hostility I earlier felt. Intuitively, it seems to me that treatment can be more effective with a willing and receptive patient. Fear can only cause all the body systems, including cell activity, to speed up and suffer from the effects of stress and surges of adrenaline.

I couldn't be a willing and receptive patient unless I could figure out a way to be in control of the treatment. Talking to my healthy cells and visualizing what was happening in my body did that for me. Meditating in the waiting room prepared me, calmed me, and kept me from having an anxiety attack every time the door to the treatment room opened.

The best side benefit of such a regimen for me was the mildness of treatment side effects. Every individual experiences side effects to a greater or lesser degree, and no one can predict who will suffer and who will not. For me, there was little or no severe nausea. A constant but tolerable "yukky" feeling became so familiar I could ignore it. My hair came out, but within a few months it began to grow back in while treatment continued. In spite of repeated warnings about susceptibility to infections I had only one—after having my teeth cleaned. Lack of energy was a problem, but gave me an excuse for saying No to extra work—something I had always found hard to do in the past.

Self-fulfilling Prophecy

"The self-fulfilling prophecy is, in the beginning, a false definition of the situation evoking a new behavior that makes the originally false conception come true. The [apparent] validity of the self-fulfilling prophecy perpetuates a reign of error. For the prophet will cite the actual course of events as proof that he was right from the very beginning."

Robert Merton, 1948

Coping with treatment and laying the groundwork for healing are enhanced by an understanding of the phenomenon of self-fulfilling prophecy. Originally defined by Robert Merton more than forty years ago,[7] this phenomenon has been repeatedly recognized and verified by psychologists. We have an amazing capability to make dreams come true—even when the dream is a nightmare. For me, it became essential that I not internalize the negative beliefs of others about my condition. I worked to replace fear words and gloomy predictions with my own words of encouragement and hope, and positive expectations of getting well. This was beyond positive thinking—it was a more fundamental restructuring of my own beliefs and my responses to others so that I would not become an unwitting victim of self-fulfilling prophecy.

As I encountered doctors and other cancer patients during my treatment, I could see that the phenomenon of self-fulfilling prophecy was nowhere more active than in cancer treatment. I had some frustrating conversations with patients. Too often they went something like this:

Me: "What kind of cancer do you have?"

Patient: (Breast, bone, prostate, colon, etc. ...)

Me: "And how are you doing?"

Patient: "Not good. The doctor has given me a year to live."

Feeling some responsibility to give hope where there seemed to be none, I would sometimes protest. How could the doctor know for sure? Hadn't there been many cases of spontaneous remission? What about the patient's own healing mechanism and will to live? How could one person's chances be determined by mere statistical probability?

The responses I received were depressingly similar. Most were angry at my interference. They did not want their faith in their doctors' prognoses to be shaken or even questioned—*even when that faith was killing them.* They defended the prognoses fiercely, bringing in additional evidence that their illnesses were indeed terminal. "I *am* dying! My doctor *said* I was dying!" It may have been the only certainty they had to cling to, and they were not willing to give it up in favor of an elusive possibility of healing.

These patients would die on schedule, thus proving their doctors correct in their prophecies and adding to the growing body of statistics that would in turn be used to predict the outcome for later cancer patients.

I developed a new theory, one which seems at least as plausible an explanation for the cancer mortality rate as any that currently exist. It goes like this:

Most people believe that cancer is fatal. More specifically, many *doctors* believe that cancer is fatal. They have statistics available to them that predict the patient will die from the disease in slightly more than half of all cases. They in turn pass on this belief either overtly or subtly to their patients. I read that message in a hundred ways from my doctors, even when they weren't saying it in words. The doctor who would not cross the threshhold of the examining room. The tone of voice, the averted gaze, the falsely cheerful note in a response. The choice of words: "Breast cancer is an insidious disease," meaning, "It will kill you later if it doesn't kill you now."

The belief of the doctors often is offered in the form of a prophecy, especially if you ask about your chances for survival. The prophecy in many cases is that it is likely you will die from the disease, because X percent of others with your particular form of the disease eventually died from it.

Patients are anxious, desperate, exquisitely alert to every communication from their doctors. They pick up every nuance, every word, and even though they may not be able to repeat the verbal message they understand perfectly what they are expected to do. Die.

The prophecy thus sets up a dismal expectation in the patient's own mind, and the patient organizes her thoughts, attitudes, and behavior around that expectation. The power of her own belief contributes to the state of her health. It becomes a squirrel cage, a particularly vicious cycle.

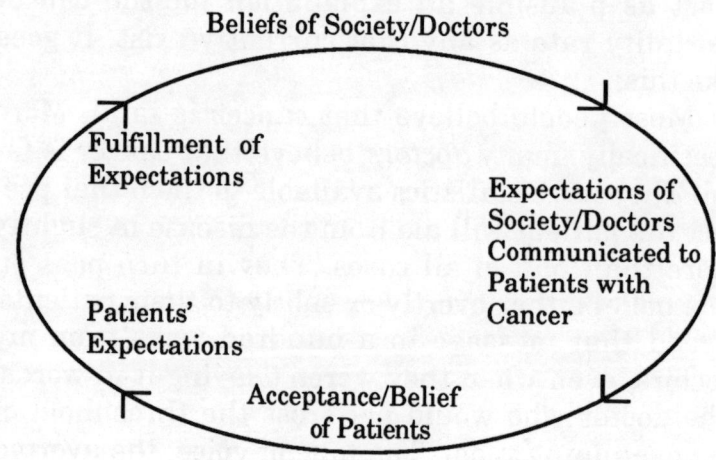

Beliefs of Society/Doctors

Fulfillment of Expectations

Expectations of Society/Doctors Communicated to Patients with Cancer

Patients' Expectations

Acceptance/Belief of Patients

The Vicious Cycle of Self-Fulfilling Prophecy

The cancer mortality statistics have not changed significantly in a hundred years in spite of many advances in cancer treatment. This may be because our *beliefs* about cancer have not changed. Patients are set up, and will probably die of cancer if they willingly accept these beliefs without question.

Regardless of any advance in treatment that may emerge in the future, unless it is so dramatic that it changes the worldwide *belief* about cancer, the overall statistics are likely to remain the same.

Self-fulfilling prophecy is a phenomenon we have all experienced personally, and scientific research has given us more evidence of its effects. Edward Jones, a Princeton professor, reviewed in *Science* magazine studies in which people attributed liberal or conservative views to other experimental subjects, even though they themselves had pushed the buttons that caused the others to read prepared statements.

In another experiment, men were assigned to make get-acquainted phone calls to women. When they were told that they were talking to attractive women, they were significantly friendlier than when they were talking to women they thought were plain. The women, who had been randomly assigned, were poised and confident in response to callers who had been led to believe they were attractive, and were tense and uncomfortable with the other callers.[8] According to this research, it is reasonable for a perceiver to act on an expectation and for the target person to be affected.

"What is not so reasonable," Jones adds, "is for the perceiver to take the other person's reactions to his own behavior at face value..." The perceiver will be more likely to continue to interpret the other person's reaction in accordance with his own beliefs and expectations. If a patient, for example, denies the doctor's perception that cancer is fatal, the patient is said to be in denial, and is counseled to move on to the next stage of dying, for his own psychological well-being.

Educators are all uncomfortably familiar with the study in which teachers were given comparable groups of students, but some teachers were told they had low achievers and other teachers were told they had high achievers. The first groups then performed below their abilities and the second groups performed above their abilities. Neither the students nor the teachers were aware of the experiment, but all demonstrated the effectiveness of expectation and self-fulfilling prophecy.[9]

However, the cycle of belief-expectation-belief-expectation-fulfillment can be interrupted, and the more often patients are willing to do it the more likely it is that the overall statistics will begin to show an increase in the survival rate.

The way to interrupt the cycle and to permanently change the system is to stop it here:

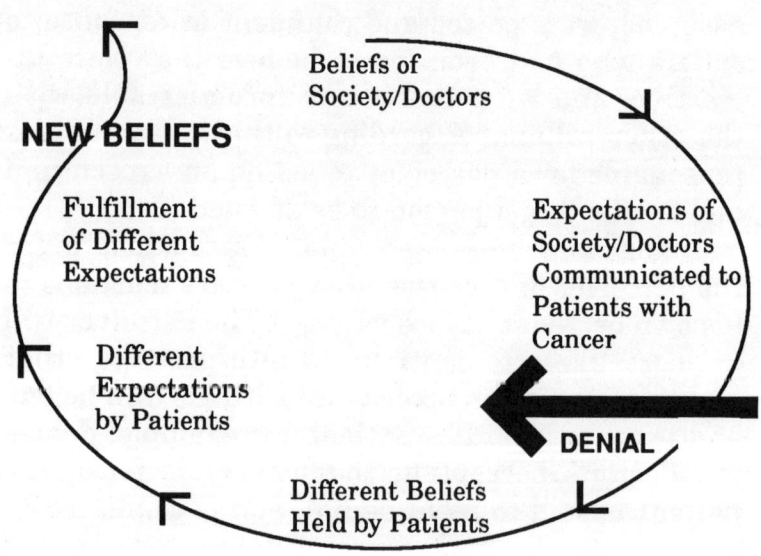

Beliefs of
Society/Doctors

NEW BELIEFS

Fulfillment
of Different
Expectations

Expectations of
Society/Doctors
Communicated to
Patients with
Cancer

Different
Expectations
by Patients

DENIAL

Different Beliefs
Held by Patients

The Healing Cycle of Self-Fulfilling Prophecy

Part of managing your treatment is to refuse to accept the negative predictions you may hear from your family and friends and from your doctors: predictions about the effects of treatment, the eventual outcome of the disease, and your own particular chances. You can ask your doctor not to use certain words that you find frightening or unacceptable. *Remission*, for example, which implies that absence of cancer is only temporary. If the word *cure* sticks in his throat as an acceptable substitute, perhaps he would be willing to use *cancer-free*. Also ask that he not modify that phrase with the words "at present," or "for now."

With your family or friends who are giving you support, decide on some words you will use as substitutes for those negative words that express uncertainties as if they were certainties. This may seem silly, but it has become apparent to me that my brain hears and processes and acts on the words that it hears, even—and *especially*—from my own mouth. It is as if the Universe listens carefully to everything I say or think, and then pours all its energy into fulfilling what it interprets to be my wishes.

For this reason, if the prognosis is "five percent chance of survival," I change that phrase in my mind to "survival is possible," and whenever the frightening number pops into my mind, I replace it with the more hopeful phrase—both are equally true, but you can choose to use the power of self-fulfilling prophecy to heal rather than to harm.

Managing your treatment will be an ongoing responsibility, but once it is underway you can turn your attention to even more important matters— marshalling your immune system to cope with treatment and to defend against cancer in the future. If you wish to be weller than well, you will need to pay attention to those factors which have an effect on immune strength and take charge of those factors. Lifestyle, emotions, thoughts, diet—all can have scientifically measurable effects on immune cells. Now you will need to take charge of your lifestyle.

---

[3] Laudenslager, M., Ryan, S., Drugan, R., Hyson, R., Maier, S., "Coping and Immunosuppression: Inescapable but not Escapable Shock Suppresses Lymphocyte Proliferation." *Science 83,* August 5; pp. 568-570.

[4] Derogatis, Leonard, "Psychology in Cancer Medicine: A Perspective and Overview." *Journal of Consulting Clinical Psychology*, October, 1986, pp. 632-638.

[5] Levy, S., Herberman, R., Lippman, M., d'Angelo, T., "Correlation of Stress Factors with Sustained Depression of Natural Killer Cell Activity and Predicted Prognosis in Patients with Breast Cancer." *Journal of Clinical Oncology,* March, 1987, pp. 348-353.

[6] Nelson, D.V., Friedman, L.C., Baer, P.E., Lane, M., Smith, F.E., "Attitudes of Cancer: Psychometric Properties of Fighting Spirit and Denial." *Journal of Behavioral Medicine,* August, 1989, pp. 341-355.

[7] Merton, Robert K., "The Self-Fulfilling Prophecy," *Antioch Review,* 1948, #8, pp. 193-210.

[8] Jones, Edward, "Interpreting Interpersonal Behavior: The Effect of Expectancies," *Science 86,* October 3, pp. 41-46.

[9] Rosenthal, R. and Jacobsen, L., *Pygmalion in the Classroom,* Holt, Rinehart and Winston, 1968

Chapter Three

Third Stage:
Taking Charge of Your Lifestyle

The Farm

*A*t this writing I live with Jack on a farm in the Coast Range of Oregon—rain country. The cedar and fir trees are hung with long pale-green veils of moss, and in the summer the woods and roadsides are overgrown with salmonberries, blackberries and thimbleberries, just as there were when I was a child. It feels like coming full circle. I grew up on a flower-bulb farm on the coast only fifty miles west of here.

The small house was crowded with five children. Family life centered around the round oak dining table in the kitchen, which my mother covered with a pretty tablecloth at mealtime. When the table was loaded with food for dinner—home-baked bread, home-churned butter, homemade jam, beef or pork or chicken we raised on the farm, several kinds of homegrown vegetables, milk, apple pie or strawberry shortcake with whipped cream—my father would beam with satisfaction and announce, "Everything on this table we produced ourselves, except the flour and salt." He spent time, occasionally, musing about how to manage the flour and salt. But wheat wouldn't grow at the coast. Too wet.

From my earliest memory we all helped with the farm work. I was the least willing farm worker of all the children. I begged to be allowed to bake the bread or clean the house instead, letting the others plant daffodil bulbs in the mud. But I never tried to dodge the work of "topping" the daffodils in the spring—pulling the creamy golden tops off the flowers so the growth energy would go into the bulbs we marketed. When I knelt between the rows in the daffodil field my mind apparently recognized the importance of that image and stamped it into my memory. I can still close my eyes and see again the eye-level sweep of sweetly swaying sunshine, butter-yellow to the horizon on all sides.

My parents were gentle representatives of the Protestant work ethic. A small family farm on the Oregon coast required a substantial degree of work ethic to survive. But the farm was also an ideal playground for a dreamy child, and there was plenty of time to create secret hideaways in which to read or dream, or hide. One such special place was a sun-dappled vestibule by the Skipanon River, down the slope from the house, arched with alder trees and floored with moss. Such peace and quietness I found there.

During the summer heat I would explore the woods across the road, building a lean-to against a large Douglas fir tree, using limbs as a frame and cedar boughs as roofing material, and bringing layers of moss to add padding to sit on. It was shadowy inside but I had learned to read in the dark. After bedtime I read by candlelight or under the covers by flashlight—until I tried to read under the covers by candlelight. The small fire instantly brought my mother's attention to the matter and the jig was up.

But I was ambitious. When it was rainy and cold or hot and dusty and the bulbs still had to be planted or dug, I amused myself by imagining the life I could have instead. Every Saturday when we made the trip to the county library I checked out five books, the library's limit. In the books I found the images of other lives. Girl detective. Journalist. Spy. Nurse in a big city hospital. New York City. Paris. Tramp steamers.

My mother, who wouldn't have the opportunity to go to college until she was in her fifties, was quietly determined that each of her children would go to college. I saw college as my way out of the small farming and fishing community literally at the farthest edge of the country.

Climbing the Ladder

Even ambitious young women in that 1950's era were aware of other expectations—fostered and fed by reading *Ladies' Home Journal* and *Good Housekeeping*, and by taking the obligatory Home Ec in high school. College at sixteen was overlaid with marriage at eighteen and motherhood at nineteen. By the time I was twenty-two I had three children, but I also had a teaching degree.

After teaching for three years, I took advantage of an opportunity to work with the designer of an educational computer. I wrote programs, sold computers, trained teachers, and developed curriculum. Before long I was caught up in the excitement of directing a federally funded computer education project.

My first marriage did not survive the strain of these major changes in our lives, and I moved with the children to Portland, to a position as senior research scientist in a research and consulting organization—another career advance. My sister lived with us and helped with the kids and the house, and I was more free to make business trips when I had to.

Three years later we moved to Iowa so I could pursue a doctorate, and I married again. Completing the degree, we moved back to Oregon, where I returned to the organization I had worked for before moving to Iowa. Soon I was transferred to Alaska, where I directed a statewide telecommunications project under contract to the State Department of Education. I loved the job—reveled in the challenge and the daily design and people problems to work out. It seemed that everything I had dreamed of had come true.

It lasted a year and a half. The state assigned a new supervisor to oversee our contract and he resented my presence. In the face of growing conflicts with him I struggled to resolve the problems, but nothing worked. He wanted complete control, and so did I. What had been a smoothly running project was now beset with obstacles. I refused to give up, trying this or that strategy to win his support, unsuccessfully.

Frustration and anxiety swirled in my mind, keeping me from falling asleep at night and waking me at three or four in the morning to begin again the endless recounting of the details of the irresolvable conflict, searching for some solution. At work I was dulled and irritable from fatigue and loss of sleep. Finally I had to give up the struggle, yield to the inevitable, and resign before I was fired.

I returned to Portland and was reassigned to a small project. In Alaska I had directed a staff of fifteen—I now had only myself, and no secretary. I had to begin again from nothing and build a program, swamped with anger at myself, anger at the circumstances, and depression. No doubt feeling lonely and abandoned, my husband began his own abandonment of me. I was too preoccupied to notice.

The Fast Track

"There is more to life than increasing its speed."
Mahatma Gandhi

My lifestyle for many years had revolved around the self-imposed necessity to raise a happy family and to achieve increasingly elevated professional goals. Money, fame and power seemed important. Working for agencies funded by grants and contracts we were always in a low-bid environment—that is, understaffed and overcommitted. When traveling I tried to schedule red-eye flights so I could put in full days at each end of the trip. Even then I often worked on the plane, trying to catch up with impossible deadlines.

Long hours, deadline pressure, and twenty years of heavy travel finally stopped being fun. My first professional failure in Alaska, the collapse of my second marriage, and the onset of cancer all brought me up short. Why had the exciting, challenging, successful golden years suddenly changed? It was time to reassess everything.

For twenty years I never really unpacked my suitcase. A veteran traveler with double cosmetics, hair dryers and toothbrushes, I kept one of everything in a small case that was always ready to go. I owned several little two-wheeled stainless steel carts, the kind with vertical racks and elastic cords to secure the bags. However, the ones I bought regularly squeezed my bags out sideways onto the floor, usually when I was running to make a connecting flight, and the wheels often came off in the middle of a trip. Fortunately most major airports have a shop which sells little wheeled carts. After studying flight attendants, who always seemed to have their bags under control, I finally discovered the kind with big sturdy wheels and industrial-strength cords.

In every major airport, I knew the best places to buy stamps or food or books or ice cream, and the location of mailboxes, automatic bank teller machines, copy machines, and sit-down phone booths. I knew how to wheedle my way onto a full flight when unexpected events left me stranded in a strange airport.

I found ways to compensate for jet lag, botched travel plans, late flights, strange cities and unfamiliar hotel rooms. I knitted a large, soft, stretchy, comforting "blanky" to wrap myself in on airplanes, which were usually too cold when they were not too hot. I carried soft slippers to wear in flight and flat shoes for sprinting through airports. Whenever possible I traveled in blue jeans, until I discovered that a well-dressed person with a ticket labeled "Dr." would sometimes be upgraded to first class.

On every flight, I worked. It was the only way to keep up with the unremitting schedule at the office, and was a welcome opportunity to catch up, or just to catch my breath. Locked in that quiet cylinder 30,000 feet in the air there were no telephones, no supervisors sounding alarms, no subordinates wanting direction or advice, no new opportunities to respond to. My most productive work was done on airplanes. When laptop portable computers became available, I was first in line. Now I could be even more productive on airplanes.

Back in the office, it was a different matter entirely. One typical day two years after my return from Alaska was memorable because by the time I collapsed into the car for the long drive home, I was absolutely certain I no longer enjoyed any part of this work, and had to find a way out. That typical day was just one day too many.

I had arrived home from Philadelphia after midnight the night before, and left for the office before dawn that morning. Another major deadline loomed—by four o'clock that afternoon we had to have twenty perfect copies of a proposal ready for pickup by an overnight express service for delivery to Washington D. C.

Everything that could go wrong went wrong. Insult piled on injury as we all scrambled to do the impossible while ignoring the intolerable. This barely controlled panic was repeated on a regular basis in my work. Early in the afternoon I paused to call and inquire about a proposal we had sent off the week before. The expensive 24-hour delivery service we used had delivered the precious package two hours late. Under the rules, it could not be accepted.

If only I had had the proposal ready a day earlier...

But I still had the proposal due out this afternoon. I would skip lunch again.

In earlier years this pressure cooker existence had been challenging and exhilarating, and I loved the creative possibilities. I thrived on the satisfaction that came with meeting an impossible deadline, balancing the needs of the staff against the needs of the organization. My co-workers and I celebrated such achievements and congratulated each other for "doing it again." I welcomed opportunities to show what I could accomplish, was proud of my ability to manage people and events, to solve problems and to constantly come up with new ideas and creations. I usually did my best work when under the greatest pressure, and I learned to expect it of myself. At these times there was certainly stress in ample measure, but there seemed no price to pay.

Gradually, things changed. Years of overdrafts against a diminishing energy account began to take their toll. My physical and emotional health began to suffer. At the age of thirty-seven, I developed high blood pressure. I had relied too much on my robust health, demanded too much of myself for too long.

Stress is inevitable in any life. Stress is change, and we cannot and should not avoid it. Most people, however, react with the fight or flight response so useful to our prehistoric ancestors and so harmful to us: deep in the brain, the hypothalamus responds to an alarm from the frontal lobe and releases chemicals, pouring adrenalin to the heart, speeding up breathing and heart rate, sending extra oxygen into the brain and lungs, and increasing blood pressure.

I had grown so accustomed to the frequent adrenalin surges that I had come to depend on them to cope with the demands of an overfull and overscheduled life. It was only after I had left that job that I realized I had become chemically addicted: I was an adrenalin addict.

Marrying Jack was a first positive step toward healthy change. Since he was also a program director we had the same pressures and responsibilities and could frequently travel together. We understood each other's hectic lifestyle. He had lost his wife of twenty-eight years to chronic lung disease, and was at the same crossroads as I—we were ready to do something about that lifestyle. We no longer felt immortal. We wanted to cherish every moment, and to make more time for the really important things.

As long as we stayed at our current jobs there would be little opportunity to slow the pace. Jack looked ahead to the possibility of retirement at age fifty-five, and decided he could easily manage the remaining four years of work. I began to look for alternatives for myself. Nothing was available that would provide professional challenge, allow a forty-hour week with no travel, *and* pay well. Perhaps I would have to modify some of those goals.

But we could do something about our personal lifestyle. Soon after our marriage we found the farm. Intending to buy a small, well-kept acreage within half an hour's drive of Portland, we instead fell in love with a large neglected farm an hour and a half away. The house was old and shabby, in need of major remodeling before it would be comfortable. But the important things were all there: a fresh and tranquil creek just behind the house, fragrant honeysuckle vines lavishly engulfing the back porch, blueberry, raspberry, loganberry, blackberry and currant bushes in the yard, rhubarb by the doorstep, a well-cultivated garden.

Evenings, an elk herd grazed in the pasture behind the woodshed. Half the land was heavily timbered. Walking back through the property with the real estate agent, I recognized from childhood the familiar dense fragrance of sun-warmed moss and felt a response of deep pleasure and peace. Jack saw a unique opportunity to build something productive and beautiful—a house that needed his carpentry skills to become a home, and land that needed his management talents to become useful. It also offered the possibility of an alternative career after early retirement. We made an offer the next day—and it was accepted.

Dog and cat came with it, and we soon added goats and horses. The long commute became a welcome chance to talk without interruption or distraction. We had three hours a day of undisturbed communication, talking about the farm or the family, comparing notes about work, planning, dreaming, laughing, learning to know and appreciate each other. The drive was lovely, through miles of unspoiled timber country. It was a needed buffer between the tranquility of the farm and the stress of our jobs. We grew to look forward to it.

Now there remained the job stress to conquer. I knew the relationship between conflict and stress, and cancer. There is laboratory evidence that stress depresses the immune system function. The attack cells of the body routinely trounce the cancer cells that are present in all of us all the time. But the number of attack cells, called immunoglobulins, actually decreases when the body is under emotional stress or conflict.

The Simontons had observed that cancer patients often experienced a major personal loss or conflict from six to eighteen months prior to the diagnosis—usually the loss of a primary relationship through divorce or death, job loss, or personal failure. For some women, it was the empty nest syndrome. Stress alone is not the key factor—it takes the stress of helplessness, of conflict that appears to offer no way out. I recognized all of these in my own life in the year prior to the diagnosis. Cancer is often the last straw in a series of personal disasters.

For me, all the irresolvable conflicts were behind me. Personal serenity seemed possible, if I could eliminate the job stress. Aware of the well-documented effect of stress on the immune system, I was troubled by fear that this stress could again compromise my defenses, leaving a fertile field for cancer to return.

When the teaching position at the university opened, I hurried to apply. By now I was fearful that a second tumor was growing, and I had relinquished many formerly important beliefs. The university salary was exactly half my previous income. I had to change my belief that the amount of money I could command was a determiner of my value.

There was little travel money available at the university, so the professional activity that kept me in the limelight would be curtailed. Could I give up the limelight? Yes—I realized that I no longer needed it to verify that I was important. In fact, relative anonymity seemed to offer a welcome respite. The most difficult adjustments would be giving up a secretary and going from a large office walled by windows to the tiny, cramped, airless cubicle available to a faculty member with no seniority. But what I gained was more control over my schedule, more decision-making autonomy, less travel, and a more relaxed academic atmosphere.

At the university there was less need for fight or flight, and at first I had trouble settling down to a predictable routine. Here I could schedule my teaching, research, and student advising. I could and did say No to requests for outside consulting or travel. I found that for several months I was restless and jumpy, expecting the alarm to sound in my brain, ready to leap into action. It took time to learn the different kind of joy, that of being proactive rather than reactive, choosing my own challenges rather than constantly scurrying to respond to the snowballing demands of the job. I had to learn to enjoy life without the exciting chemical addiction of adrenalin.

In my entire career I had never taken a coffee break. I knew it would be possible at the university to leave the office without telling anyone, saunter two blocks to a coffeehouse, and enjoy a cup of coffee while reading the morning paper for half an hour. In fact, as a professor I seldom find time for this glorious pleasure, but it is enough to know I can *choose* to take a break whenever I please.

By the time the second cancer was diagnosed, the stress in my life was on its way out. Family, home, and work conflicts had been resolved in favor of peace. The only significant stress that remained was that of having cancer. That stress would have to be addressed in a different way—by taking charge of my thoughts and attitudes.

A Personal Miracle: Your Immune System

*"That the universe was formed by a fortuitous con-
course of the atoms, I will no more believe than that
the accidental jumbling of the alphabet should fall
into a most ingenious treatise on Philosophy."*
Jonathan Swift

No one knows what causes cancer. It is believed
to be a combination of things: genetic susceptibility,
environmental factors, perhaps a virus, combined
with a temporarily depressed immune system
which is too sluggish to effectively attack multi-
plying cancer cells. We can do little about the first
three contributing factors, but the most important
factor, fortunately, is one we *can* affect.

The body is gifted with a remarkable, powerful,
exquisitely complex, magical and mysterious ability
to resist disease and to heal itself. Studying the
way it works one cannot help but feel amazement
and awe. That such a delicately balanced system
could be disrupted or enhanced by our emotions has
always made sense intuitively, and psychological
research indicated that indeed it was true. Now,
through the new science of psychoneuroimmunology, the evidence exists at the cellular level.

In laboratories nationwide, studies are
providing an increasing pool of research results
documenting the dramatic effects of the emotions
on the physical functioning of the body.

Norman Cousins, author of *The Anatomy of an
Illness*—the book that began the debate—has
described his own informal experiment using
himself as a single research subject: he had two

blood samples taken five minutes apart, using the first sample as the baseline. For the next five minutes he tried to put himself in a mood of joyous determination, almost celebration as he describes it. He tried to imagine what a wonderful planet we would have if the United States and the Soviet Union had rational foreign policies. He tried to imagine what would happen if these nations realized they were dealing not with bombs but with human beings, and tried to put their emphasis on their responsibility rather than just their power; on their understanding rather than their tempers.

He began to feel excitement as he imagined the outcomes of this rational approach—how we might be able to divert resources that are now going into making the planet unsafe and unfit for human habitation into a planet that can perhaps exceed its known wonders. He found himself becoming progressively excited and joyous and after five minutes he gave the signal for the second blood sample. Both samples were run through a phlocytometer which can actually measure and count the immune cells.

They found a fifty percent improvement on all the categories of cells—the NK (natural killer) cells, suppressor T cells, the cytotoxic T cells, and a 200 percent increase in the number of antibody-coded T cells—in just five minutes.[10]

While this is not a scientifically valid study, since there was only one subject, similar research is proceeding nationwide. Experiments with "the biology of hope" will lead to a dramatically altered understanding of disease and healing.

The Battle of the Robot Cells

The immune system in its complexity can perhaps be described with a metaphor. Imagine that you live on the tiny but beautiful planet Immunos, which is populated with one trillion White Robots, all of whom have been programmed with one purpose—to protect you from harm. On Immunos, you are free to wander as Adam and Eve in the Garden of Eden, supplied with all your wants and needs, and oblivious to the activity of the population of White Robots, who are eternally vigilant to care for you.

The sentry robots, or Phagocytes, constantly patrol the paths and roads, alert for foreign invaders. Sometimes affectionately referred to as "cell eaters" by the humans because they will eat anything, the huge Phagocytes also serve as a cleanup patrol, picking up and eating any debris they encounter in their continual circuits of the planet. As the first line of defense, they will try to kill invaders before they have a chance to multiply, by surrounding and eating the alien cells. The sentries are efficient and swift, unless they are overwhelmed by too many alien invaders at once.

If the Phagocytes find themselves outnumbered, a second class of defense robot is activated, the T-Team. The T-Team is a specialized class of robots programmed at the Thymus Gland Training Center. Each member of the team is programmed to perform a specific function:

T Lymphocytes:	recognize invaders
Helper T:	advance guard spies
Killer T:	seek and destroy
Natural Killer:	kill cancer cells and viruses
Suppressor T:	end the battle when it's time

The first ones to be called in are the T Lymphocytes. These robots have the unique ability to recognize the precise identity of the alien invader, through the chemical markers which uniquely identify every cell in the universe. These robots are programmed to recognize more than a million different molecular invaders that are foreign to the planet Immunos. Since T-Team robot cells can reproduce when an invasion threatens, the Lymph Node Cell Factories are put on alert at the first sign of trouble.

While the T Lymphocytes are hurrying to the invasion site, they call to their advance-guard spies: the Helper T cells. These robots have been watching at the invasion site and now leave for the Lymph Node Cell Factories with specific information about the enemy, to order the production of Killer T robot cells. The Killer Ts are programmed to seek and destroy specific viral or cancer cell invaders that have been identified by the Helper T robots.

While at the Lymph Node Factories, which are strategically placed all over Immunos, the Helper Ts also make contact with another specialized defense robot—the B Lymphocytes. B robots reside in the factories, waiting for information about invaders to begin production of chemical weapons called Antibodies which are programmed to destroy a wide range of disease-producing aliens. Production of Antibodies may take a few days, but once these weapons are completed they are rushed to the invasion site to help the Phagocytes and Killer T robot cells in their fight. The robots know the urgency of this battle—the robots must destroy the invaders before they can reproduce and attack the humans the robots are programmed to protect.

Should the invader be a cancer cell, an important first strike defense system immediately comes into play: the Natural Killer cell. This mercenary robot does not need to wait for the Helper T messengers in order to be activated. It is ready to respond at every moment to a virus or cancer. In fact, the Natural Killer cells are the most important defense against aliens of the Cancer variety. Produced just for this function, they are the mercenaries of the robot force.

As the Antibodies, the Natural Killers and the Killer T robots wage the war, the Phagocytes continue to eat aliens and to clean up the debris of the battle. As soon as it is clear that the war is being won, another member of the T-team, the Suppressor T robot cell, is called. The Suppressor T releases chemical messages that slow down and finally halt the other robots. The newly-produced robots and antibody weapons, however, will remain circulating on the paths and roads of Immunos, vigilant against the return of that specific type of alien. These robot cells, now called Memory T and B cells, act as an early warning system to give the soldier robots a head start, bestowing immunity against specific viral or bacterial invaders.

However, even protected by the wondrous White Robots, our immune systems sometimes can be overwhelmed by invading cancer cells. The immune system can be compromised by environmental factors, diet, stress, emotions, and beliefs. Most of these we can control. Even when we feel most trapped by unavoidable conflict, there are options and escape routes, if we are willing to be open-minded.

Stress and Wellness

At a symposium of the American Academy for the Advancement of Science in December, 1970, Dr. Thomas H. Holmes, a professor of psychiatry, presented the surprising results of studies spanning more than two decades: if in the period of a year your husband dies, your daughter elopes with a man you hate, and because of financial problems you have to sell your home, move into an apartment, and get a job, your chances of getting sick are eight out of ten. If on the other hand you have a year in which your husband recovers from a serious illness, enjoys unprecedented financial success which allows you to move into your dream house, and your daughter marries a man you adore, your chances of getting sick are...eight out of ten.[11]

It is simply change, regardless of the type of change, that causes sickness. According to Dr. Holmes, it does not matter whether you are the type of person who enjoys change, or whether the changes you experience make you happy or sad, or whether a particular change is socially desirable or undesirable. A sufficient amount of change, Dr. Holmes claims, leads to increased susceptibility to illness. The immune system simply lets down its guard in the face of an overwhelming amount of stimulus and challenge.

In the last ten years there has been increased interest in the notion that cancer may be partially caused by the emotions. The research has taken two divergent but related paths: to support the premise that stress and/or conflict weaken the immune system and thus decrease a person's ability to fight cancer; and to identify a cancer personality similar to the Type A personality that some believe is more prone to heart disease.

o   o   o

Stress/Immune System Research: Many studies, with animals and with human beings, have documented the effect of stress on the ability of the immune system to function competently. R. C. La Barba, in a 1970 study, reviewed all of the existing literature about stress and malignancy in animal experiments. He found that in every study, stress apparently facilitated the onset and spread of cancer. The explanation most often proposed was that stress inhibited antibody production, disturbed the hormonal balance and cellular metabolism, and upset the endocrine system—all physical disturbances which had been repeatedly linked to cancer in other experiments.[12]

New techniques and new instrumentation have spurred research in this area, with increasingly interesting results. Dr. Robert Ader, a researcher at the University of Rochester Medical Center, underscores the difficulty of implementing such research with its complex interacting elements. Given the psychosocial environment in which human beings live their lives such research requires the collaboration of scientists in many fields—psychology, immunology, endocrinology, neurology, biology, and sociology. Nevertheless, the research has begun. Psychoneuroimmunology (defined by Ader as "operating from the premise that mind and body are indivisible") has begun to take on legitimacy as a scientific discipline.[13]

If one accepts the idea that stress predisposes one to disease, including cancer, then it seems reasonable to suppose that some stress-burdened personalities may be more susceptible to cancer.

o   o   o

Cancer Personality Research: Although there is a great deal of current research relating personality to the development of cancer, there is no way to definitively make the cancer personality connection. Barrie Cassileth, a University of Pennsylvania psychologist, carried out a study in 1985 with cancer patients in intermediate or advanced stages of the disease, and found no link between attitudes and length of survival or remission. As Dr. Cassileth points out, "Cancer is an overwhelming biological event." She notes that there is a tremendous number of things happening in the tumor, the immunological and hormonal responses, and the effects of age and cancer treatments.[14]

It is useful, nevertheless, to think about the possibility of personality and attitudes contributing to development of cancer, because they are factors over which we can exercise some control. No blame or regret is necessary, just a simple recognition that we have the power to affect the outcome. We can improve the functioning of our own immunological and hormonal responses by working on attitudes and emotions as well as reducing the level of stress in our lifestyle.

The cancer personality research is therefore interesting for what it can lead us to change, certainly not as another reason to feel at fault, guilty, or to blame for the illness. To the extent that we recognize our own personality patterns that might have contributed to cancer, we also can recognize the incredible power of our emotions over our bodies, and use that incredible power to reverse the effects we have experienced in the past.

In his book *You Can Fight for Your Life* Lawrence LeShan has presented his conclusions from a twelve-year study of 450 cancer patients who were given extensive psychological testing. Dr. LeShan found four characteristics in a majority of the patients: loss of an important relationship prior to diagnosis of cancer, inability to express hostility, tension over the death of a parent (often early in childhood), and a basic attitude of helplessness and hopelessness.[15]

Other studies have confirmed LeShan's observations about the helpless, hopeless attitude of cancer-prone individuals. Drs. A. H. Schmale and H. Iker observed in their female cancer patients a kind of hopeless frustration about some conflict in their lives for which they saw no resolution. This conflict often occurred approximately six months prior to the cancer diagnosis.[16] In my case, the irresolvable conflicts in my career began nine months prior to the diagnosis, and my primary relationship began to disintegrate a few months later.

Dr. W. A. Greene studied leukemia and lymphoma patients over fifteen years, and observed that, for women, the loss of an important relationship, particularly the mother's death, was a significant life history element. Menopause or change of home were also important changes. For men patients the most significant life history events were loss of the mother, loss or threat of loss of a job, and retirement. Dr. Greene concluded that the despair and hopelessness brought on by such events contributed to development of leukemia or lymphoma.[17]

In 1987 the results of a long-term study on cancer and personality were reported. Over thirty years ago, researchers used accepted personality tests to develop personality profiles of nearly a thousand physicians in medical school. They grouped the subjects into five personality clusters and followed them for over thirty years. The lowest cancer rate—less than one percent—was in the group characterized by acting out and expressing their emotions. The highest rate of cancer—over sixteen times as high—was in the group characterized as loners who suppressed their emotions. The personality trait common to most of the clusters with higher cancer rates was a tendency to hide real feelings, particularly negative ones.[18]

Dr. O. Carl Simonton and his (now former) wife, Stephanie Matthews Simonton, have documented similar conflicts and patterns in their patients' lives, and have identified five steps of a psychological process that frequently precedes the onset of cancer.

1. Experiences in childhood result in decisions to be a certain kind of person. Usually, the kind of person the child decides to be is one who is always good, pleasing, and cheerful, suppressing any hostile feelings.

2. The individual is rocked by a cluster of stressful life events. The critical stresses that often precede cancer are those that threaten personal identity: loss of a spouse or loved one, job loss, retirement, or loss of a significant role.

3. These stresses create a problem the individual does not know how to deal with. The problem is not caused by the stresses and conflicts alone, but by the inability to cope with the stresses with the rules for behavior the patient has adopted early in childhood. The feeling of being trapped, helpless, of having no way out of the conflict comes from the limited coping resources imposed by those early decisions.

4. The individual sees no way of changing the rules about how he or she must act and so feels trapped and helpless to resolve the problem. Most of the Simontons' patients acknowledged that there was a time prior to their illness when they felt helpless, unable to solve or control problems in their lives.

5. The individual puts distance between himself or herself and the problem, becoming static, unchanging, rigid. While seeming to be coping with life, the patient may feel that life seems to hold no further meaning, except in maintaining the conventions. Serious illness or death provides a way out, or perhaps at least a postponement of the problem.

It is important to understand, the Simontons point out, that this process does not *cause* cancer, rather it permits cancer to develop by interfering with the immune system and possibly, through changes in hormonal balance, by leading to an increase in the production of abnormal cells.

The purpose for pointing out these possible relationships is not to create guilt or blame but awareness. If you recognize a similarity in your own patterns, you can intervene in the process and make positive changes to eliminate the sources of conflict and hopelessness. You may wish to find a trained counselor to help you reverse the cycle that has culminated in cancer. The important thing to recognize is that the spiral of hopelessness that may have contributed to your illness need not continue—you can change the rules you have lived by, and can change your thoughts and beliefs.

The Simontons outline four psychological steps they have observed in those who reverse the spiral:

1. With the diagnosis of a life-threatening illness, the individual gains a new perspective on his or her problems. Illness gives the person permission to change, to say no, to express hostility.

2. The individual makes a decision to alter behavior, to be a different kind of person. With the rules suspended, suddenly new options appear.

3. Physical processes in the body respond to the feelings of hope and renewed desire to live, creating a reinforcing cycle with the new mental state.

4. The recovered patient is "weller than well." When patients have actively participated in a recovery from cancer they often feel healthier than what they considered "well" before their illness. They have a psychological strength, and a new feeling of control over their lives.[19]

For those who are not yet sick, but who recognize the patterns of stress, irresolvable conflict, and helplessness in their own lives, it is possible to reverse the patterns before illness strikes. You may recognize your own fast-track lifestyle and your own personality in these descriptions, and see the danger signs in time to change. Cancer, heart disease, or some other serious illness can certainly give one the needed motivation to change one's lifestyle, but you can choose to use a more gentle approach and perhaps forestall illness entirely by making the changes in time.

Strengthening Your Immune System

Although many factors may contribute to development of cancer—genetic susceptibility, exposure to carcinogens in the environment, viruses, depressed immune system—a most important factor is the immune system. A properly functioning immune system can overcome the effects of genes, carcinogens, and viruses.

We all know of cancer-prone families, and suspect a genetic weakness that leads to development of the disease in one form or another. Yet in these same families there are usually some siblings who live cancer-free to a healthy old age. Didn't they have the same genetic history? Or were they simply able to overcome the influence of their genes? (And of self-fulfilling prophecy—seeing one's parents, brothers and sisters die of cancer can be lethally convincing.)

We all eat and breathe carcinogens daily, smoke, lie in the sun—yet only one in four gets cancer. Again, the condition of the immune system

114

at a time when cancer cells are active may be an important factor.

Fortunately, the immune system is one element over which we have direct and immediate control.

Of all the factors that keep the immune system functioning properly—diet, rest, exercise, peace of mind—the most important is peace of mind. Inner peace. The holy grail for all of us, yet more available than we imagine.

Yes, diet is important, but less important, I believe, than has been trumpeted in magazines and news reports. It may be that the power of self-fulfilling prophecy has turned good food into poison in our minds, and it then functions as poison. Because every individual is unique there can be no single cancer diet, guaranteed to protect you or cure you.

Follow your intuition about what to eat—pay close attention to what makes you feel good and energetic and well. Eat that. You learned in school about the food groups and vitamins, and you learn in daily headlines about the importance of a low-fat diet, limiting caffeine and alcohol, drinking plenty of water. Use good sense, eat when you are hungry, *enjoy* every bite, stop when you are full, and don't worry about your diet. Worrying messes up your peace of mind.

Exercise, in spite of the hype of recent years, is not the holy grail either. It can and does, however, help keep the immune system healthy. It can also contribute to your peace of mind. I have found that a brisk walk in the morning after meditation leaves me with a relaxed alertness and peacefulness along with the feeling of exuberant energy and glowing good health. Most studies with humans have found that exercise releases chemicals in the brain—

endorphins—that act as natural opiates to calm and cleanse the mind. This is probably the source of the so-called runner's high reported by runners.

Rest and sleep are essential to maintenance of a healthy immune system. Again, however, pay attention to how you feel. If you always wake up feeling rested after six hours of sleep, that's enough sleep. If you wake up groggy and tired when the alarm goes off, you need to go to bed earlier. Nothing, however, can interfere more with your ability to rest than an unpeaceful mind.

Regardless of how irresolvable a conflict or a stressful situation seems to be there are always options available if you are only willing to allow yourself to look for them. It may require that you give up some of your most dearly held convictions or assumptions. It may require listening to your intuition, your inner voice, and following its advice.

My conflict with the state's supervisor in Alaska seemed irresolvable. It kept me awake nights for months before I was willing to let go of my belief that I had to finish what I had started, that I had to succeed, and that my project was mine alone to complete. The conflict in my failing marriage was resolved once I was able, again, to let go of my belief that I had to finish what I had started, that I had to succeed, and that I was the one who had to make it work. Leaving my fast-track work life behind became possible as soon as I could give up the belief that my salary level was an essential indicator of my worth as a human being.

In every case the irresolvable conflict that was robbing my peace could have been resolved months earlier if I had recognized that the real obstacle was simply my own assumptions and beliefs, rather than anything inherent in the situation.

Perhaps these conflicts seem tame to some. What if there is a drug-addicted child, or a bankruptcy, or loss of one's home in a fire or flood, or a child or spouse with a dreadful incurable disease? Even in cases such as these people have found they can choose peace. The pain in each situation is in part from our appropriation of another's problem or pain, or our belief that we cannot be peaceful or happy or safe without that home, or that job, or that person. Yet, many have found that peace is available to them even in these painful circumstances.

In the case of a drug-addicted child, for example, we may have to release the belief that we are bad parents if the child is addicted, that we are thus responsible for fixing the problem for the child, and the belief that the child is not capable of doing it for himself. All of these beliefs deny the child's own integrity or wholeness. It is that essential integrity that we must trust, and release the child to it.

The way out of an irresolvable conflict is to turn ninety degrees and take another look at assumptions you had thought unchallengeable. The most viable solutions to a difficult problem often lie in the discard pile of "things I couldn't possibly consider."

There are many ways to alleviate the effects of ongoing daily stress. Planned vacations are more important than we realize. At least two consecutive weeks a year away from work are recommended by psychologists for mental and emotional health, as well as frequent weekends of fun and play. New music is available that is specifically designed to quiet the mind and promote relaxation. Massage is wonderfully soothing, and a half-hour professional massage costs no more than half an hour working out in a health club. Exercise is a stress-releaser. The method I have found to be most useful for long-term relief from stress, however, is meditation.

Finding Peace

"An active mind is a sick mind.
A quiet mind is a healthy mind.
A still mind is Divine."

Jerry Jampolsky

Meditation need not be a formidable mental discipline. It does not require mantras, concentration, particular postures, breathing regimens, or commitment to a belief system. It is, most simply, a quieting of the mind. Some can find such a stillness at the center of the mind by running, some by fishing a quiet stream, some by praying. Many find, as I did, that meditation is a useful way to find peace on a daily basis.

My particular way of meditating is simple. Years ago, I learned transcendental meditation. The T.M. Movement had taken on the trappings of a pseudo-religion, but the technique was useful to me even without the philosophy. At that point in my life I rejected the presence of God in any form but was looking for a way to relax and release the effects of stress. Meditation was the most promising technique I could find. For a few years I practiced it on an irregular basis, and found it helpful during hectic times—if I could make the time to do it. Had I established a routine of seeking peace for a few minutes in each day, perhaps things would not have grown so frantic.

I was given a mantra by the T.M. teacher, two meaningless syllables to repeat in my mind while allowing thoughts to disappear. I no longer use a mantra because for me it seems just another way for my mind to stay active. Using imagery also keeps my mind too active, although others might find imagery or a mantra useful.

Now meditation has become a routine. I meditate each morning as soon as I awake, sitting up in bed and allowing thoughts to gradually slow down and become quiet. As I relax my muscles and let go of bodily tension and tightness, I find thoughts or worries coming back—which is a good sign. As muscles relax, they release energy, and this is experienced as bursts of thought. I allow those thoughts to blow away like leaves in a breeze. The rest of the day can be occupied with thoughts and worries—this is my time to be free of them.

I have no goal in meditation, no purpose other than to allow my mind to be still. When thoughts are persistent, I give gentle attention to the breath moving through the bridge of my nose. I don't *concentrate* on the bridge of my nose, but simply attend to it quietly, to let go of thoughts. Often, when the busy thoughts and worries finally drift away I am able to hear my inner voice, distinct from my usual "mind trash" in its quietness and clarity. I recognize it by the feeling of peace it brings, and I listen.

Training my mind to meditate is sometimes like training a hyperactive puppy to settle down and be still, to Sit and Stay. I must, first of all, seriously intend for the dog to be still. I can't simply give him the command and wander off, thinking of other things. I must stay with him and keep eye contact, keep the intention. If I walk away and he begins to scoot toward me or jumps up, I have to return and remind him, return his focus to what it is he is trying to do.

Likewise, my mind loves to scoot away in thoughts, or to jump up and rampage. Then it simply needs to be reminded that, for right now, I am not thinking busy thoughts, I am becoming quiet.

Once I have become quiet, my thoughts change. If I have a problem, a highly creative solution will often occur to me, one I could not have found in my busy, thinking, reasoning, imagining mind. These thoughts are clearly different from mental busy work. I recognize the difference by the feeling of peace that accompanies such thoughts, as opposed to the tightness in the solar plexus that accompanies mental busy work. The presence of these thoughts might be called intuition, or creative inspiration, or it might be called listening to my higher Self.

I have often used the awareness of that inner wisdom deliberately, to solve problems. I follow four simple steps to hear my creative voice more clearly:

1. *Get quiet.* Although I use meditation, one could take a long bath or a quiet walk, if that is what allows one to still one's thoughts and be at peace.
2. *Express the desire.* I express my desire to have an answer, quietly, in my mind. I say it once and let it go. It need not be repeated.
3. *Listen.*

4. *Expect an answer.* It helps to have paper and pencil ready to write down the answer, because that expresses my expectation of an answer.

There are times during meditation when I realize that time has passed but I was not having thoughts. These are the moments of absolute stillness and peace that are called *transcending* in Transcendental Meditation, and *the holy instant* in *A Course in Miracles.* In these moments, however brief, we are in touch with the Infinite.

In the silence of meditation we find our peace. That is where we hear our quiet inner voice, that part of the mind that knows the truth, our higher Self. Believe it. I recognize that voice as familiar, a whisper I have heard since my earliest childhood memory, before the more strident, aggressive, accusing voice of ego drowned it out.

If prayer is asking for help perhaps meditation is listening for the answer. Too often we ask the question or make the request but are not listening when the answer is given, so we do not hear it.

For me, the holy grail was as close as my own mind. When I learned to be quiet, still my mind, and listen, I found the inner peace that was waiting for me there in that tranquil place. The higher Self, that part of the mind that is always involved in creating, knows the answers to all problems.

During a busy day if I stop for a moment and pay attention to my thoughts I find a jumble of little scraps of fear in its many forms: defenses, judgments, accusations, worries, lists, deadlines, strategies, plans, guilt...

If I can take a brief time-out to relax my body and quiet my mind, the scraps of fear fade and disintegrate. In that inner peace I hear the truth which is always the opposite of the fear thoughts: safety, orderliness, love. The perceived threat is seen as illusory, the perceived attack is seen as merely a call for love, the strategic planning is seen as unnecessary.

Whether you seek inner peace in running, enjoying nature or in meditation, the more you practice listening the more clearly you will hear that quiet, truthful inner voice. The holy grail, inner peace, is as near as your own mind in your own quiet place.

---

[10] Cousins, Norman, unpublished address to the Tenth International Congress of Hypnosis and Psychosomatic Medicine, Toronto, Canada, February, 1986

[11] Holmes, T. H., and Masuda, M., report to a symposium of the American Academy for the Advancement of Science, Dec., 1970

[12] LaBarba, R.C., "Experimental and Environmental Factors in Cancer," *Psychosomatic Medicine*, 1970, 259

[13] Ader, Robert, "Clinical Implications of Psychoneuroimmunology," *Journal of Developmental and Behavioral Pediatrics*, December, 1987, pp. 357-358

Ader, R., Cohen, N., Felten, D., "Brain, Behavior, and Immunity," *Brain Behavior Immunity Journal*, 1987, #1, pp. 1-6

[14] Cassileth, Barrie, quoted in Baker, G.H., "Invited Review: Psychological Factors and Immunity," *Journal of Psychosomatic Research*, 1987, #1, pp. 1-10

15 LeShan, Lawrence, *You Can Fight for Your Life: Emotional Factors in the Causation of Cancer*. Harcourt Brace Jovanovich, Jove Books, 1977

16 Schmale, A.H., and Iker, H., "Hopelessness as a Mediator of Cervical Cancer," *Soc. Sci. Medicine*, #5, pp. 95-100

17 Greene, W. A., "The Psychosocial Setting of the Development of Leukemia and Lymphoma," *Annals of the New York Academy of Sciences*, 1966, #129, pp. 794-806

18 Shaffer, J., *et al.* "Clustering of Personality Traits in Youth and the Subsequent Development of Cancer Among Physicians," *Journal of Behavioral Medicine*, 1987, #5, pp. 441-447

19 Simonton, O. C., M.D., Matthews-Simonton, S., and Creighton, J. L., *Getting Well Again*. Bantam Books, 1980

Emmett Fox has said:

*"I am not my mind,
I am not my body,
I am not my emotions...*

I am spirit...

*I am a divine individualization
of God."*

Chapter Four

The Fourth Stage: Taking Charge of Attitudes

A Bad Attitude

---

*B*y the time the second cancer was confirmed I definitely had an attitude. I was crouched in a defensive position, smiling through clenched teeth, angry at the disease, the doctors, the prognosis, the treatments, well-meaning friends. My anger was fueled by a feeling of betrayal that the visualization techniques I had earnestly followed had not led to a permanent recovery. Not only was I sick, but now, with what I had learned about the mind-body connection, I was weighed down with guilt that somehow I had not managed to keep the correct thoughts, and thus had directly contributed to, if not actually caused, the present catastrophe.

Worse, I suspected the guilt was justified. Knowing the effects of stress on mental and physical health, I had nevertheless clung for a time to a marriage that was over, attempting to fix it and prolonging the agony and the stress. Rather than finding ways to ease the pressure of my job, I concentrated even more intensely on work as a way to forget the marital problems. No doubt, I reasoned, those months of unusual stress after the first cancer was a time in which the second cancer had ideal conditions in which to grow. It was my fault. I was to blame. And my guilt was appropriate. Yet I found some relief in the knowledge that I could also blame my former husband for putting me through those months. My anger at him, finding this new fuel, rekindled.

However, the betrayal by my first oncologist gave me the clearest focus for my anger. Hadn't he misled me about the potential risk in my experimental treatment? Hadn't he ignored the symptoms of a new tumor? Hadn't he then given me a death sentence with no emotion at all? I nursed these injustices and recounted them to others, comforted by their reactions.

I was fully involved in several of Elisabeth Kubler-Ross' stages, certainly anger and depression. Radiation and chemotherapy depleted my energy and made depression harder to fight.

One woman, a good friend to me and to Jack, knew of my belief that one's thoughts can influence one's health. She frequently sent me sunny "Have a Nice Day" cards with cheery notes. In spite of her good intentions, the cards enraged me. I felt vulnerable, judged, exposed in my failure to achieve health with positive thoughts. I wrote about those feelings in my journal:

July, 1983

Terry is today's rage target. This morning she told me with a big smile of a dream she had last night: I was sick and Jack asked her to move out to the farm—MY FARM!!—and "take care of things." INCLUDING HIM?? In her dream she did move to the farm and took care of the farm and Jack too, while I was too weak and sick to participate. Telling me of this (to her) delightful dream, she was oblivious to my indignation and outrage. AMBULANCE CHASER!! HEARSE CHASER!!

Terry's cards and notes all have the same relentless message: Chin up! Cheer up! Think positive! Keep smiling! LET HER GET CANCER, PLEASE GOD, AND SEE IF SHE KEEPS SMILING.

Terry and I have talked about the importance of a positive attitude. I know her message is that I brought this on myself with my inability to manage my life, with my anger and loss and flailing. I don't want to hear it, especially from a woman who dreams of taking over my farm and my husband. Especially with that gnawing feeling inside me that says she is right, that I did bring it on myself. And Jack could do worse than marry Terry if I die.

OVER MY DEAD BODY!!

o   o   o

Anger, guilt, fear and depression. Those emotions dominated my life for a few months. I found an outlet for the anger at my first oncologist by initiating a malpractice suit. The malpractice attorney I worked with was eager to pursue the case. He had a relaxed confidence that we would win. I spent hours poring over medical charts and finding evidence to support my case. While it gave me an outlet for my anger, it did not diminish it.

I was suffering. I tried to change my attitudes, terrified that I was digging myself a deeper and deeper hole, depressing my immune system and thereby cancelling any remaining small chance of getting well. But it was impossible to change—I could not pull myself up by my own bootstraps. Floundering in that quicksand of anger and guilt and debilitated by treatments, I felt incapable of becoming positive. What was there to be positive about? So-called positive thinking seemed a trivial and inadequate technique for dealing with serious, life-threatening and overwhelming situations. It seemed to be the conceptual equivalent of the sappy and tiresome happy face symbol—easy to use when times are not too tough, but worthless for the heavy duty problems.

It was at this low point that I took another look at the set of books I had purchased a year earlier, called *A Course in Miracles*. I had heard it described as "self-administered spiritual psychotherapy," and that certainly seemed to be in order now. Reading the Introduction and browsing in the Text and the Workbook, I realized that the *Course* is about healing. The key elements in healing, it said, are forgiveness and replacing fear with love. It defined only two emotions: love and fear. Anything that is not love is fear. Guilt, then, is fear? Yes. At bottom, guilt is fear. It made logical sense. Anger is fear? I thought about the things that made me angry. If the layers of righteous justification were peeled back, there was nothing left but naked fear. Fear of dying, ultimately.

The *Course* had a single purpose: to "undo" the belief structure that is based on fear, guilt and anger which leads to misery and sickness, and then to begin to build a new belief structure based on love and forgiveness, and which leads to joy, peace and healing.

It seemed like a tall order, but I could no longer bear my state of mind. I was ready, now, to begin to work on my attitudes. This *Course* felt like the right tool for that work. The Workbook of the *Course* offered 365 lessons, one a day for a year. I could take ten or fifteen minutes to do one every morning.

The first few lessons made me feel foolish. They are intended to undo the belief that our perceptions of the world represent reality. After practicing the exercises with each lesson for two weeks, I felt so silly that I quit. The lessons seemed to present an upside-down view of the world. However, the Text maintains that the world we *perceive* is the one that is upside down. I wasn't as ready to change my attitudes as I thought I was. This was too extreme for me to accept. Changing my beliefs about the world seemed like brainwashing.

A few more months went by, with no relief from fear, guilt and anger. I decided to give the lessons another try.

The concept of "God" came up early in the lessons. This definition of God was different than the one I had earlier rejected: God, according to this

129

Course, was not vengeful and was not separate from me. God is my Source, and my mind is part of God's. Perhaps I could accept the word God as long as that definition was a part of it. This God is a god of love, of forgiveness, who accepts and loves me exactly as I am. A paragraph in the text became a comfort I turned to again and again:

"How can you who are so holy suffer? All your past except its beauty is gone, and nothing is left but a blessing. I have saved all your kindnesses and every loving thought you ever had. I have purified them of the errors that hid their light, and kept them for you in their own perfect radiance. They are beyond destruction and beyond guilt. They come from the Holy Spirit within you, and we know what God creates is eternal."

A Course in Miracles, Text, p. 76 (First edition)

The concepts that I had to understand before going on in the *Course* were those of *ego* and *higher Self.* Ego is defined as that part of the mind that believes it is separated from God, and perceives everything in the world from that frame of reference.

It is this thought or belief of separation from God that is beneath sin, guilt and fear, and builds a thought system based on attack to protect itself. It is this part of the mind that constantly tells us that we are in danger. It knows only fear. We can think of the ego as a tiny circle inside a much larger circle which represents our higher Self. Both circles are made of the same stuff, but the ego has put up a barrier of beliefs and lies and seeming limitations

130

to keep us from being aware of our true, unlimited nature.

We spend most of our time enclosed within the belief structure of that little circle, seeing a world of pain, punishment and attack through its distorting curtain. We can press against the seeming limits of the circle by constantly challenging our beliefs, challenging the ego's view of the world—and begin to see glimpses of the truth of our spiritual nature.

When the ego bombards us with negative and fearful messages about ourselves and others, we can challenge our beliefs by choosing to listen to the opposite message, the message whispered by our higher Selves.

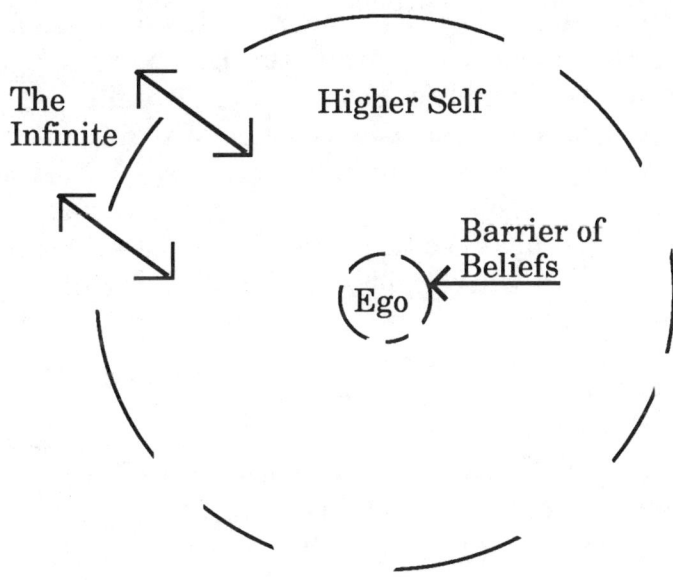

The Illusory Barrier

Our higher Self is our spiritual mind, that "still, small voice" that we all recognize as the truth. It is the part of our mind that knows only unconditional love. It does not recognize attack, guilt, or anger.

The word *sin* is not used in the *Course*, except to redefine it as simply *error*. If we are children of God, and we are doing the best we can and learning and growing why should our mistakes be called sins and be punishable by death? I thought about my own children, learning to walk and falling down again and again, but improving with each new try. Would I punish my child for her mistakes in learning to walk? Of course not. Would God punish his children for mistakes? Not likely.

I gave the *Course* a serious effort now, spending the first quarter or half hour of each day in study and meditation, trying to incorporate the lessons, trying to undo the belief structure, the ego structure, that had brought me so much pain. I saw little progress at first. It was especially difficult to practice forgiveness. Forgiveness, however, was the key to healing, so apparently I was going to have to do it. Forgiveness seems to be the key to all forms of healing, in all religions and belief systems. I would not be able to avoid confronting the importance of forgiveness.

Some of these lessons were tough.

"I am not the victim of the world I see."
"God's will for me is perfect happiness."
"Forgiveness is the key to happiness."
"If I defend myself I am attacked."
"In my defenselessness my safety lies."

Talk about upside-down thinking. I was unwilling to try to test these concepts except in small ways. I tried being defenseless in a conflict with an angry student. Instead of meeting hostility and accusation with hostility and counterattack, I simply allowed the student to express her anger and agreed with her, and resisted the urge to defend myself. She finally apologized and said that perhaps she had jumped to a wrong conclusion. I didn't have to say a thing. Could it be that defending oneself in the face of a perceived attack actually intensifies the attack? Could this principle work in more important areas?

I tried to forgive, starting with my former husband. I succeeded. Several times. It was like quitting smoking. The more often you quit, the better you are at quitting. But a few weeks later, there is the cigarette in your hand.

Finally I realized that forgiveness, rather than being an instantaneous one-time release is more like melting an iceberg. The tip of the berg represents the thing to forgive, the obvious injustice. When you have successfully forgiven the person you blame for this injustice, the iceberg appears to have vanished. You feel lighter, freer, happier—until a few weeks later, when a random event or thought will push a button that triggers a memory, and you realize the iceberg is back. Again and again you forgive, melt the iceberg, and feel freer.

This iceberg seems indestructible. Each time you forgive, a new part of the iceberg floats to the surface, and you have to do it all again. This continues to happen until you realize that you are not letting go of the same frozen resentment over and over, but that each melting down reduces the size of the berg, and allows a new portion of it to surface and to be melted. And finally, the day comes when you realize that it is truly, forever gone. The button is still there to be pushed but all the wires have been disconnected. Your memories no longer cause pain and anger.

The Workbook lessons continued in what I recognized as a spiral curriculum. That is, there were only a few essential concepts to grasp, but they were repeated again and again, at increasing levels of complexity. When we teach a child in kindergarten to do arithmetic, we only teach the number symbols, and how to count. By fourth grade they are using the symbols to do long division, and in high school to do calculus. This *Course* was progressing in a similar spiral.

Gradually, the beliefs that governed the way I saw the world were being dismantled and gently replaced with new beliefs. Love in place of fear. Safety in place of danger. Forgiveness in place of cherished grievances. Freedom in place of guilt. Healing in place of sickness.

Brain washing indeed. Mind cleansing.

It was becoming clear to me how I had made myself sick. Guilt was unnecessary, because making myself sick was not a sin but simply an error born of ignorance. I had demonstrated to myself the incredible power and strength of my own mind, and now I could choose to reverse that power and use it to heal my mind and my body instead.

With daily study, meditation, and practicing of new behaviors and thought patterns, I was noticing some new phenomena. Miracles. Daily miracles. They were easy, natural, and totally effortless.

I was developing a new habit of listening to my higher Self rather than to my ego and found it a more certain way to operate. People I would have expected to be hostile were instead eager to please. Attacks turned into conversations. Tasks that should have been difficult were quick and simple. All my relationships, even those with people no longer in my life, were healing. I was beginning to be aware of my thoughts much of the time, and was shocked to realize how often those thoughts were based on fear or judgment. The next step was to change the thoughts, reverse their direction, and exchange fear and judgment for love and forgiveness.

I dropped the malpractice suit, to the bafflement of the attorney who was making good progress and was certain of winning. My reasoning was simply practical: in the two years that it would take for the case to come to court, I would have to hold onto my anger and my conviction that I had been seriously damaged—that I would probably, in fact, die because of a doctor's negligence and ethical lapses.

To continue the lawsuit my thoughts would have to remain unforgiving and defensive—attack thoughts. If I were to be convincing in the courtroom, I would have to *believe* that I had been harmed and would probably die. I would have to remember and recite every particle of evidence demonstrating that I was in serious trouble because of this doctor's mistakes. My heart wasn't in it. I no longer had a wish to punish him. Moreover, by now I was certain that my mind would believe its own story and would scramble to grant my wishes. There was no longer a need to sue. I had not been damaged.

A growing sense of peace told me I was on the right track. In spite of continuing treatment and dire predictions from doctors, I was actually happy.

Chemotherapy ended after nearly two years and I faced a very different future than the one I had contemplated for so long. Everything seemed possible. I had new tools to work with and was certain that I had indeed healed myself. Medical treatment was one of the tools I had used, but the energy and effort I had put into *spiritual* healing, it seemed to me, was the key. There was no doubt in my mind that I had successfully practiced four stages of getting well—choosing to live (denial), and taking charge of my treatment, my lifestyle, and my attitudes—and was now cured of cancer.

Was there a fifth stage? My inner voice told me that there was, but it was unclear to me what it might be. Healing of the mind, perhaps? Or wasn't that simply part of stage four, taking charge of one's attitudes? Never mind, I would start writing the book about the stages of getting well anyway. Cured of cancer, I had a story to tell.

Mind-cleansing Techniques

Anger, guilt, fear and depression. All are emotions, or ego-reactions, that interfered with and even sabotaged my efforts to get well. They seem to be impossible to overcome, keeping one's mind captive and scrambling desperately in an endlessly revolving squirrel cage.

These are the emotions that depress the immune system. These are likely to be the emotions that set up the conditions in which cancer could get a foothold in the first place, and the inability to get rid of them increases the frustration and guilt.

I had to find ways to let go of such emotions, even before I could see any good basis to feel hopeful or happy. Wallowing was okay for a while, and I followed the guidance of counselors who recommend really feeling the emotions, giving myself permission to feel lousy until I was sick of feeling lousy. I certainly did that. But when I was ready to feel better, I needed some techniques to help change my direction.

For me techniques alone were never enough—I always needed to understand the reasoning and the belief underlying the techniques. Yet, I did know that sometimes real change comes from "acting as if." One of my children recently reminded me of a suggestion I had made when she was small: when something is hard to do, just do it until it gets easy. She used that in her life on many occasions. Sometimes the understanding and the belief come after the fact. Just a little willingness to try to change, a little willingness to understand is enough.

Practicing these techniques or any others demonstrates your little willingness and opens the door to change and understanding. It is taking the first small step with which any long journey must begin.

Cast Out Fear With Love

"Fear and love are the only emotions of which you are capable."
    A Course in Miracles, Text, p. 202 (First edition)

What are the attitudes that contribute to disease and create obstacles to healing? You can answer that for yourself, if you pay close attention to what makes you feel bad, and what makes you feel good. There may seem to be a complicated array of emotions—frustration, anger, anxiety, depression, helplessness, guilt, blame, indignation—and we can always place the responsibility out there on someone or something outside ourselves. Seldom can we find genuine relief from those emotions, however. We are told by some counselors that expressing the emotions will allow us to let them go. Sometimes that works. Often it seems to lead instead to an escalation of the distress.

If we give some quiet thought to the complex array of emotions that cause the distress, we can identify the source: love or fear. If it is fear, we can be sure the emotional response is simply ego-reaction. Sometimes the specific fear takes some work to pin down, because we are accustomed to denying the real source of negative emotions. But if we persist, we find the truth: if it isn't love, it is fear. And all fear is merely a *call for love*.

Fear and love cannot co-exist.

The technique for transforming any negative emotion, then, is to replace the fear with love:

• • • Trace the emotion to its root. Get to the bottom of the emotion: identify as clearly as you can the fear which triggered the emotion.
• • • State the belief that underlies the fear.
• • • State the *opposite* of that belief.
• • • Consciously choose to replace the belief with its opposite.
• • • Consciously choose to replace the fear thought with its opposite.

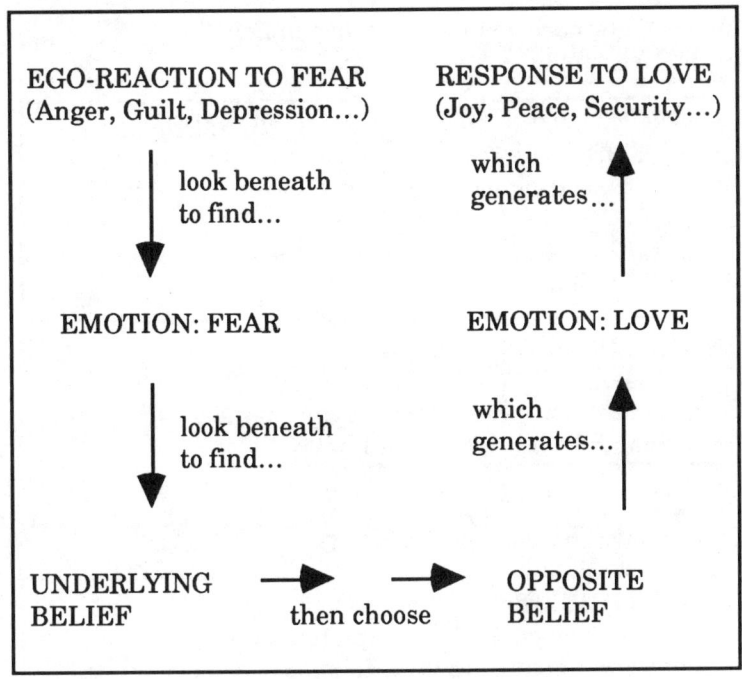

EGO-REACTION TO FEAR
(Anger, Guilt, Depression...)

look beneath
to find...

EMOTION: FEAR

look beneath
to find...

UNDERLYING
BELIEF

then choose

RESPONSE TO LOVE
(Joy, Peace, Security...)

which
generates...

EMOTION: LOVE

which
generates...

OPPOSITE
BELIEF

Replacing Fear With Love

Some examples might be useful here, from my own experience.

After the delivery service failed to deliver our proposal by the deadline, my supervisor used me as a bad example for the other program directors at the next Division meeting. Although it seems trivial and unimportant now, at the time I was furious at him and at myself, feeling guilt as well as anger. Tracing those emotions of anger and guilt back to their roots might look like this:

> EGO-REACTIONS
> Anger: "How dare he humiliate me publicly?"
> Guilt: "Why was I so incompetent?"

> EMOTION UNDER THE EGO-REACTION: FEAR
> (messages from the ego)
> "What if my colleagues agree that I was incompetent?"
> "What if I WAS incompetent?"
> "What if I lose the respect and love of my colleagues?"
> "What if I lose my job?"

> BELIEFS UNDER THE FEAR
> "I am in danger."
> "I am competent only if my colleagues agree that I am."
> "I am valuable and safe only if I have this job."

I could have chosen opposite beliefs:

> OPPOSITE BELIEFS
> "There is no danger that can threaten me."
> "I am as I was created to be: intelligent and competent."
> "What anyone else thinks of me is none of my business."
> "I am as I was created to be: valuable and safe."

> EMOTION UNDERLYING THE BELIEFS: LOVE
> (messages from the higher Self)
> "My supervisor is afraid. He is afraid he will appear to be
> incompetent because of my failure. He is afraid he IS
> incompetent. He is afraid he will lose the respect and love
> of his colleagues. He may be afraid HIS supervisor will
> publicly humiliate HIM. He is afraid he may lose his job.
> He believes he is in danger. His apparent attack is really
> only a call for love."

> RESPONSE TO THE AWARENESS OF LOVE
> "I am at peace and utterly safe. Instead of walking out of
> the meeting I will react with affectionate humor to respond
> to his call for love and to ease his fear and my own."

Reversing the Cycle

An everyday example might be the rage we feel when an inattentive driver cuts us off in traffic. The ego reacts with messages of fear: "I could have been killed!" "Who does he think he is?" "Now I'll be late for work!" The underlying beliefs are that we are not safe, that the action of the other driver truly threatened us, that we have rights that were violated. What would the opposite beliefs be?

Repeat these steps every time the thought reappears. Be dogged. You *can* restructure your beliefs and thus your emotions, but it takes vigilance and determination. You have spent a lifetime with these thought-habits, so it may take a little time to reverse them. It is like dismantling a brick house, brick by brick, and rebuilding it in an entirely new form. Gradually you will see the changes become habit, and a new way of thinking and responding will be a part of you.

It helped me to have the *Course* to study, to articulate the beliefs that I wanted to change. The ideas I was encountering did not seem new; I recognized them as truth I had always known in my deepest Self but denied at the conscious level.

You may find that a caring psychotherapist or an insightful friend can give you the support you need as you work to reverse the beliefs and habits that you recognize as leading to pain and sickness rather than to joy and peace and wellness.

Regardless of the support system you choose, however, it is essential to recognize that you have the answers *within you*. Whatever ideas, concepts, or beliefs you encounter, including those in this book, you should check out with your intuition, your higher Self, your deepest knowing. Do you recognize it as true for you? How does your solar plexus feel when you contemplate the idea? If it's a tight, tense feeling like the one you get when the roller coaster starts its plunge, that is fear. It is not truth. If you feel peace instead, that is love, and it is truth, and you should pay attention to it.

Your higher Self knows only peace, joy and love. Your ego knows only fear, and constantly tries to mask the reality of the peace that is always present by throwing up a static shield of fear.

Forgiveness

"Forgiveness is the bridge between illusions and the truth."

A Course in Miracles, Workbook, Lesson 134

Forgiveness is the source of healing. Forgiveness is release, freedom, a reversal of all you had thought undeniable—that you were wronged, betrayed, harmed. Forgiveness recognizes that you were not harmed, so there is nothing to forgive. Forgiveness dissolves guilt, releases anger, and lifts depression. Like pushing a rock uphill, when you finally, wearily reach the mountaintop your arms are suddenly light, and the rock rolls away unbidden. Forgiveness transforms. It transforms you and it transforms the world you see.

Whether a culprit deserves to be forgiven is irrelevant, regardless of the enormity of the crime. You deserve to forgive. You deserve the healing you will experience when you have released yourself from the chains with which continued condemnation binds you.

I gradually realized that my main task in getting well would be to learn to forgive. I would have to forgive injustices long treasured, forgive thoughtless oversights and deliberate cruelty, forgive strangers and loved ones, and finally, forgive myself. It seemed an impossible task, but I was willing to try. And a little willingness is all that is ever necessary.

The *Course* provided several lessons on forgiveness, and techniques to accomplish it. The tecniques were helpful, but I was not successful at first. I was still holding out, reserving out certain special grievances or special people who were beyond forgiveness. Yet, the gifts forgiveness gives were mine only when I managed complete forgiveness. I would have to keep working on it.

A major iceberg in my mind was the injury that I believed had been done to me by my former husband. I forgave Bruce again and again only to find that a grievance was still there. I wished him bad luck. Then I earnestly meditated, visualized him as happy and well, and forgave him. But some time later something would trigger an old hurtful memory and the grievance would feel as fresh as ever.

Again I would meditate and visualize him as a friend to whom I wished happiness and good fortune, someone who had enriched me by being in my life. There were times when I felt it was uselessly spending energy—I was only going over the same ground again and again, taking two steps forward then two steps back.

Once I heard a news report about a pickup truck being struck by an airplane on a runway in the city where Bruce now lived, and had an immediate flash of vengeance—"Let it be his pickup"—followed by another flash of shame and guilt for having such a horrible, irrational thought. More meditation, more forgiveness.

Finally, after years of this seventy-times-seven forgiveness, the day came when I realized it was all done. There was finally a deep certainty that I would never cherish those grievances again. The persistent forgiveness had paid off. Now there was one more thing I needed to do to finish it: tell him. I sat in my office on a quiet morning, got his office telephone number from Information, and dialed it immediately.

Without rehearsal, I simply said what I had to say: "I know you probably have been feeling guilty for years about what happened, and I'm calling to let you know that it's unnecessary. I was not harmed in any way. I am whole, healthy, and happy. I trust you are, too. The worst we did was to make mistakes. The mistakes did not matter, because we are unharmed. There is nothing to forgive because no harm was done. We are innocent, both of us."

Bruce was stunned speechless with my call, and obviously touched. His voice was choked when he finally said, "You can't know what a load of baggage I've been carrying. Thank you for calling." And then we chatted for a few happy minutes about his children and mine, catching up, and wished each other well. We had not spoken for years and have not spoken since, but when I hung up the phone I was joyous. I felt free, light, and unexpectedly absolved of my own guilt. In the years since the phone call I have found no further need to forgive him, or myself for my own mistakes in the marriage. There truly is nothing to forgive.

Forgiveness is necessary only because of condemnation and judgment. If we had never judged a person, or perceived an action as a sin, forgiveness would not be necessary. My parallel task, as I learned to forgive, was to learn to withhold judgment so that forgiveness would not be so necessary in the future.

Forgiveness is practiced instantly whenever there is a temptation to judge, as well as practiced regularly to release old grievances. Lesson 134 in the *Course* suggests a simple way to forgive:

> "When you...are tempted to accuse someone of sin in any form, do not allow your mind to dwell on what you think he did, for that is self-deception. Ask instead, 'Would I accuse myself of doing this?'"

I tried this. Just asking the question redirected my perceptions. It put me in the other person's shoes. I found I am much more likely to forgive *myself* of the very indiscretions, oversights or insults for which I judge others, because I know my own motives. I know what good intentions, weariness, frustration, or simple inattention lie behind my own affronts to others. I am more willing to give myself the benefit of the doubt.

I found to my dismay that the grievances I cherish the most and am most unwilling to forgive are usually the very same ones I have committed myself against others. On the surface, at least, I could rationalize the acceptability of my own behavior more easily than that of others.

Another question to ask when struggling to forgive is, "Have I never been in need of forgiveness myself?"

From my journal:

Someone suggested an experiment, and I tried it: List the five "sins" that I find hardest to forgive. Be specific— name names, name the specific wrong that was committed in each of the five cases. Then relax, keep an open mind, and objectively scrutinize the list. I found that I recognized on the list the very "sins" I have committed against others. In fact, they were the "sins" I have felt most guilty about, most defensive about, and for which I most needed to forgive myself.

How can I forgive myself? It helps me to recall the passage from the Course, "God remembers every good and kind and gentle thing you have ever done, and He never knew about the rest." It is impossible for God to see me as anything but what I am: sinless, guiltless, His creation. Would I accuse, judge, or condemn my child for stumbling as he learns to walk, or for making mistakes when learning to talk?

I am learning the truth about myself, that I am one with God. It is a difficult thing to learn, and I make mistakes. But God is gentle and kind, and sees me only as His beloved child. He sees me as learning, growing, making mistakes, but innocent in His sight.

If forgiveness is the most important thing we need to learn in this life, it is the hardest to do. While we are trying to uncover the deepest layers of hurt and anger from the past and to forgive the events that caused them, we are at the same time experiencing today's hurts and anger, which will become our struggle to forgive in the future. It seems we take a step forward when we forgive the past, then find that the present has become the past and we take a step backward again to deal with a new batch of things to forgive. How can we cut short this endless cycle of experience—>judgment—>condemnation—>anger—>forgiveness?

I started to notice that there seemed to be, for me, several *levels* of difficulty in forgiving.

If the forgiveness can begin before the event has taken on "reality," it is much easier, lighter, quicker. When we are not daily creating new things to forgive, the future is left blessedly peaceful.

The trick is to release the event immediately, before it is processed by the brain and sent into long-term memory. Thousands of things happen in our lives each day, and we remember only a fraction of them. Unfortunately, that fraction is often made up of the negative, hurtful things. These are the things we have processed, analyzed, rehearsed, recalled, retold, and cherished until they have taken on a rock-hard reality for us. Now we have a long-term forgiveness task.

How to release immediately? Ask yourself, "Would I accuse myself of this?" Or, "What is the call for love that I am seeing?" Or, "How does God see this person?" Or use the question my mother often asked when I was a child fretting or anxious over some circumstance: "Will this matter fifty years from now?"

To the extent that I could release perceived sins from my judgment as soon as they occurred, I was cleansing my mind and freeing it for the future. Those perceived sins that I allowed to become "real" in my mind became icebergs, to be forgiven only through repeated efforts, "seventy times seven."

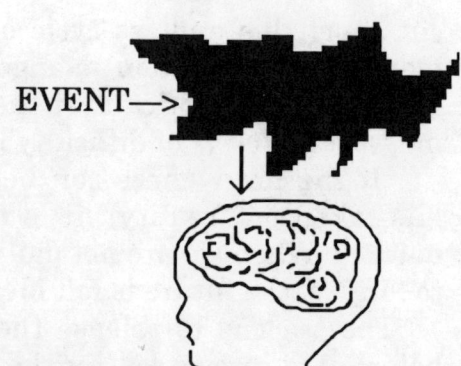

EVENT—>

FIRST LEVEL

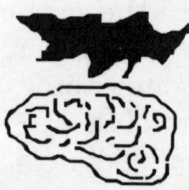

The event has just happened and I can choose to let it go immediately—to pay it no mind. Only a slight impression is made on my consciousness.

SECOND LEVEL

I validate and reinforce the "reality" of the event by harboring the memory, analyzing, attributing emotions to others, and thinking of what I should have said or done. A deeper impression—the beginning of a groove— is made on my consciousness. The event takes on "reality."

THIRD LEVEL

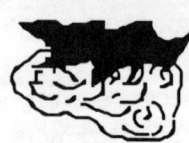

I tell someone about the event, embellishing and reinforcing its "reality" by getting someone else to agree that I was harmed. The groove is getting deeper.

FOURTH LEVEL

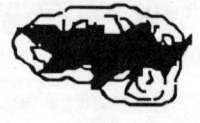

I frequently remember the event with resentment, bitterness, anger and hurt. Now I have a serious "Something to Forgive." I've worn a deep groove in my consciousness with the memory of the event.

Levels of Forgiveness

Anger

The most useful purpose that can be served by anger is to help you recognize the fear or the guilt within yourself that you are projecting onto someone else. The ego will want to work through the anger by justifying it, expressing it and sustaining it. You always have the option, instead, to choose to let it go—to recognize the illusion and to simply let it go. It will usually require you to forgive, and to reverse the thoughts you are having about some other person. When you feel stuck with the anger give it to your higher Self to manage and neutralize for you. Whenever it returns, give it back to your higher Self to deal with. Gradually you will realize that the anger is gone.

But—never feel guilty for the temporary measures you use for temporary relief while you are learning to heal. If you need to express anger, do it, and let it go—without guilt. Expressing anger to feel better is a temporary measure, expression of an illusion to relieve an illusion. It is what you use until you can let go of anger *without* expressing it.

When you do decide to express your anger, pay attention to how you feel before, during and after, in your mind and in your body. Do you feel better? Does the feeling last? Then remind yourself that the source of your anger—the cause of it—is an illusion. It is projection. Express it if you must, but then ask yourself what it is you are projecting.

Some of the research on the link between attitudes and cancer seems to suggest that a way to prevent cancer is to express one's emotions, to give in to anger, to recognize when you are feeling anger, anxiety, despair and depression, and not to repress such emotions. Yet, there are two ways "not to suppress" negative emotions: express them, or transform them. Emotions can and should be fully experienced and released. Negative emotions such as anger and depression, however, can be *transformed* rather than expressed in attacks on others, which only intensifies our distress.

Peace Pilgrim, a woman who spent the last twenty-eight years of her life on a cross-country walking pilgrimage for peace, suggests the following as a way to deal with anger:

"Tremendous energy comes with anger. It is sometimes called the anger energy. Do not suppress it: that would hurt you inside. Do not express it: this would not only hurt you inside, it would cause ripples in your surroundings. What you do is transform it. You somehow use that tremendous energy constructively on a task that needs to be done, or in a beneficial form of exercise."[20]

Try washing all the windows, or going for a brisk walk or run, or mowing the lawn with a manual lawnmower. Bake bread and knead it by hand. Weed the garden. Let the anger energy be transformed into something healing.

Depression

"When you are sad, know this need not be. Depression comes from a sense of being deprived of something you want and do not have. Remember that you are deprived of nothing except by your own decisions, and then decide otherwise."
A Course in Miracles, Text, p. 57 (First edition)

Depression is the most difficult emotion to overcome. Pulling yourself up by your bootstraps, I discovered, seems to be impossible when your boots are sunk to the hips in a quicksand of depression. Depression, however, is a normal response (albeit an ego-reaction) to some of life's disasters. At bottom, depression may be repressed anger, anger turned in on oneself, and beneath the anger there is always simple fear.

My depression after leaving Alaska was repressed anger at the people and the circumstances I held responsible for my failure, and mostly at myself. And beneath that anger was fear—that without constant, visible achievement and success, I would have no identity, no wholeness.

Even more repressed was my anger at my husband's emotional abandonment, and beneath that the fear of another failure and of aloneness, and if my partner left me, of loss of my wholeness. It is said that women tend to use depression or sadness to mask anger, and men tend to use anger to mask sadness. In my case it was true.

Depression is an attack on yourself, self-hatred, a complete identification with your ego, your lower self. The way to overcome depression, then, is to

151

recognize it as ego-identification and reverse the process. Turn to your higher Self, go within to find peace and, finally, joy. Deny the denial of truth. The truth about you is that you are safe, whole, complete and sinless, and you deserve to give yourself a break. Forgive yourself. Allow yourself to feel your complete safety. Even if your depression is from the loss of a loved one, distinguish between grief and depression, and allow yourself to feel the cleansing purity of grief without the self-judgment or anger or fear that causes depression.

Perhaps if I had been consciously aware of and had access to my higher Self in 1979, I would not have remained in a long depression, and perhaps would not have developed cancer. During that time, I did not meditate and did not realize the importance of finding a way to connect with a universal, unalterable truth about myself and about all others that would lead to peace and joy rather than to anger and depression.

When you change your thoughts, you change your experience of the world. You can always choose joy. You are free to decide to experience joy rather than depression. You can choose the beliefs and thoughts you will hold in your mind. You can learn to monitor your thoughts and notice when they take a negative turn. When that happens you can consciously and deliberately choose to replace a negative thought with its exact opposite, silly as that may seem to you at the time.

All of this takes practice and we are all capable of learning it. When it is practiced with steadfast determination the rock of depression settled in your mind will gradually begin to break up and disintegrate. You will begin to notice joy replacing depression spontaneously.

Guilt

"All healing is release from the past."
    A Course in Miracles, Text, p. 240 (First edition)

Gerald Jampolsky, a physician and psychiatrist, has written a helpful book, *Goodbye to Guilt: Releasing Fear Through Forgiveness*. Jampolsky founded the Center for Attitudinal Healing in Tiburon, California where catastrophically ill children and their families learn to find love, joy and peace of mind in place of sickness and despair. He defines guilt as, very simply, the feeling of self-condemnation that we experience after we do something we think is wrong. Guilt and fear are related and frequently synonymous. The purpose of Jampolsky's book is to show that the healing of relationships—the most important issue that all of us face in our lives—can be accomplished through forgiveness, by saying goodbye to guilt and letting go of the fear and blame that keep us separate from each other.

Relationships can be healed, Jampolsky says,

1. When we let go of guilt and fear through forgiveness,
2. When we have peace of mind as our only goal, and
3. When we learn to listen to our inner voice as a guide for directions and decision-making.[21]

Guilt is a useless emotion. It can not repair the past, but only serves to perpetuate and reinforce the past. It is an illusory concept, a creation of the ego that reminds us constantly of our sins and demands punishment. The exercise of forgiveness is nowhere more important than in releasing ourselves from guilt.

We are free to choose to be ego-slaves, slaves to and victims of our ego perception of the world, and suffer the pain of anger, anxiety, fear, depression, and guilt. Or we can choose to press against the seeming limits of that little circle of beliefs in which the ego attempts to imprison us. In choosing to see beyond the ego's limited belief structure, we will see the truth of who we really are.

---

[20] *Peace Pilgrim* , Ocean Tree Books, Santa Fe, New Mexico, 1983, p. 64

[21] Jampolsky, Gerald G., M.D., with P. Hopkins and William Thetford, Ph.D., *Goodbye to Guilt: Releasing Fear Through Forgiveness.* Bantam Books, 1985

Chapter Five

Working on Stage Five

A New Tumor

By the summer of 1985 I was beginning to feel triumphant and even smug. Chemotherapy had ended in January, a year earlier than my oncologist had predicted, and I was now seven months beyond it, a magic figure for me. The doctors had made it clear they expected a "rebound relapse" soon after the chemo ended—surely within three months. Well...then absolutely by six months. Still clean. Okay, well, this is encouraging, and unexpected, maybe we can go for a whole year. Maybe we should quit making predictions.

I was beginning to feel smug indeed.

We planned a three-week vacation for August and September, in our new/used R.V., and I began to scribble notes for the book on the stages of healing.

Before leaving on vacation I kept a routine appointment for an annual followup exam with my radiologist, Dr. Roberts. As he examined my breast, misshapen by surgery and hardened by radiation, he slowed and pressed until I complained that it hurt. He nodded.

"Do you examine your breasts?" he asked me.

"Oh, from time to time," I answered. I didn't, much.

"Feel that?" I was reluctant to feel where he was indicating. "It's about the size of a kidney bean."

Yes, I felt it. It was (Oh God) hard. When my fingers touched it, there was the familiar sizzle of fear, quickly controlled. We had a conversation about mammograms and how soon I was to see my regular oncologist, Dr. Paul. Middle of September, six weeks away.

"Don't worry," he said calmly, as he sent me on my way. "But have a mammogram right away and see Dr. Paul."

I protested. "Both times before, the mammogram has shown nothing, even right before surgery. Why bother?"

He was firm. "But this time might be different. Have the mammogram. This is a hard, fixed growth; a mammogram would confirm the need for a biopsy."

Don't worry. Right.

Twelve days later I kept a routine appointment with Dr. Michaels for my annual surgery followup. I didn't tell him what Dr. Roberts had found. I waited as he examined me. He frowned. "Do you examine your breasts?"

Oh God.

"Please lie down," he directed. More probing. "Here, see if you can feel this." I could. The hard little kidney bean was still there.

"So, what are the possibilities?" I asked him.

"Well, cancer of course."

"What else?" I asked.

"Maybe scar tissue," he suggested. I could see he didn't believe it was scar tissue.

"I want to biopsy that," he went on. "We'll do it in the outpatient clinic. Tomorrow."

"No. I don't want a biopsy, not yet. Give it some time. Let's watch it. If it's scar tissue, it won't grow." I was sounding like the doctors I had been so angry with for telling me over and over, "...let's just watch it for awhile."

"Let me work on it for a while by myself," I proposed.

Dr. Michaels frowned. He didn't like this. I was feeling in control, but he was uncomfortable. "Well, O.K., a few weeks—not a day longer. Then we'll do the biopsy."

I bargained for time, and promised to come back for a biopsy in a month if my own methods didn't work. I was unwilling to climb back on the cancer carousel and start it all again. More than unwilling, I flatly refused. Their methods clearly had not worked. Why try them again?

It was time to call on the new belief system I had so carefully built over the last months and years. The methods of medicine had failed, not once but twice. Surgery did not cure me. Radiation did not cure me. Chemotherapy did not cure me. All that these treatments had accomplished was to postpone what appeared to be inevitable, and at great personal cost. The medical establishment could do little for me.

Even so I had placed more trust in their beliefs than in my own beliefs. The scientific method dictates that one believes only what one has evidence to support. I had no evidence now to support the belief that medicine could cure me. Yet I had not given much faith to anything beyond medicine. It was time to try another method.

Preparing for Stage Five

As we prepared to leave for three weeks in the Grand Tetons, I was frustrated and scared and puzzled. I thought I had figured out the five stages of getting well, or at least the first four. I had certainly begun to take charge of my treatments, I had changed my life style dramatically, had taken charge of and changed my attitudes— so what was it that I hadn't yet understood? Perhaps it was stage five, still fuzzily taking shape in my consciousness, that I was to learn now.

Part of it was already clear: *to heal the body, one must first heal the mind.*

I had been working on that. But there must be a final stage of healing of the mind that I hadn't mastered yet. If I could understand the final stage, it might be the key to getting well and staying well.

The Tetons would be a good place to learn it. The vacation would be a blessed respite, a chance to spend full time on healing.

My way of learning this imperative lesson would be threefold, I decided: reading/study, journal writing, and prayer/meditation. I packed my worn copy of *A Course in Miracles*, a box of other books, and my portable computer and printer. I was accustomed to meditating, so that would be easy. Prayer, however, was still a problem for me. I never had understood what prayer is, exactly, or how to do it. When God seemed distant and not friendly how could one talk to God comfortably?

Learning to Pray

A few nights before we left I had trouble sleeping and dug out a book about prayer. It seemed a good time to try to better understand how to pray, not something I do easily or well. My prayers were inarticulate mumblings inside my head or heart, not well-put or neatly begun or neatly ended. My praying has always seemed to me like slipping a note under the closed door of heaven.

This book on prayer quoted I Thessalonians 5:17, "pray without ceasing." I recalled an astonishing scene, witnessed years ago in Mexico City at the Shrine of Guadalupe: hundreds of pilgrims crawling to the Shrine for miles on knees worn, lacerated and bleeding, in pitiful supplication and devotion.

How could God require me to beg on bloodied knees for what I want or need? Why should I have to pray without ceasing that I be healed? Does God want me to beg, so that He can then finally, grudgingly, grant me that which I seek? I resisted and resented this notion, refusing to *beg* God to heal me. My heart sent out little protestations, "No, wait!" My heart wanted to beg. I didn't let it.

The next morning, still frustrated at my inability and unwillingness to pray for healing, I had an experience that became a watershed for me: I heard for the first time my own inner voice, the voice of my higher Self. That comforting and loving voice let me know that there was no formula for prayer, and no necessity to beg. I recorded it in my journal:

August 17, 1985

This morning I woke, read the daily lesson in the [Course in Miracles] Workbook, and meditated for awhile. Deep in meditation, no thoughts in particular, a phrase (possibly a Bible verse I'd heard as a child?) popped into my head, as if it were being spoken by a voice from inside me. It was so clear, set apart from the background noise in my mind, spoken with conviction. The words bell-like come to mind. The message was:

"Your prayer was answered before you spake it."

I was flooded with joy at this message, recognizing immediately that it was true. No bloody knees necessary here. This had to be God speaking to me. It sounded like a Bible verse—I'll try to find it later.

I've always wondered how it sounds when God talks to you, envied people who have experienced it, wondered why he didn't talk to me, too. Or maybe he had spoken to me and I was busy elsewhere, or didn't listen, or didn't

160

understand. For years I had sought to clearly hear an inner voice, but seemed to hear only my own thoughts. This time the difference was distinct. If this was my own thought, it came from a different source than I was accustomed to hearing.

Happy and comforted, I went to find Jack. He was leaning against the kitchen sink, his favorite place to smoke and read. "God spoke to me!" I announced.

"He did?" Jack looked up, eyebrows raised. "What did he say?"

"He told me, 'your prayer was answered before you spake it.'"

Jack dragged on his cigarette and tried hard not to laugh, but didn't succeed.

"What's so funny?" I asked. "Doesn't God ever talk to you?"

"Sure he does."

"Well," I persisted, "what does he say?"

Jack laughed again. "Usually he says, 'listen you stupid shit.' Not once has he ever said 'spake.'"

So maybe God speaks to you in your own words. Maybe the message I heard was a Bible verse I remembered subconsciously from childhood. Maybe God is, as the Course *maintains, the source of my true Self. My higher mind. My unconscious? Why should God be unconscious? How can I make him my conscious mind?*

o   o   o

This journal entry reflects my growing awareness that prayer had a place in my spiritual growth, and that prayer was not necessarily a one-way outpouring of pleas, demands, and confused questions. Nor was prayer even necessarily articulate; it didn't even need words. And, the answer was given as soon as the need was felt. A

161

little book, *The Song of Prayer: Prayer, Forgiveness, Healing* gave me more insight:

> "Everyone prays without ceasing. Ask and you have received, for you have established what it is you want."*

I believe that every thought is a prayer, even when it is without words, and every prayer is answered.

I found an exhaustive concordance to the Bible, and looked up "prayer," "spake," and "answered." There is no verse similar to the message I heard so clearly, although there is one which seems close:

> "It will also come to pass that before they call, I will answer; and while they are still speaking, I will hear."
>
> *Isaiah 65:24*

The journal entry on prayer ended with this:

"Your prayer was answered before you spoke it," sounds like I have already seen the end of this movie, but now I have to stay in the theater and sit through all the drama and bloody battles to see how it gets to that perfect ending. The tumor is still there, but I know it's only the beginning of the movie. And I already know how it will come out.

o   o   o

---

* *The Song of Prayer: Prayer, Forgiveness and Healing.* Foundation for Inner Peace, Box 1104, Glen Ellen, CA 95442

A few days before we left for the Tetons, my daily Workbook lesson gave a gentle promise:

Lesson 131: *"No one can fail who seeks to reach the truth."*

This was reassurance that, indeed, I had already seen the end of the movie.

On the Road

The R.V. quickly came to feel like home, comfortable and snug, away from telephones, television, work, and interruptions of any kind. I had a goal for this trip: to discover stage five, and to heal myself of the new cancer.

The journal entries during the trip reveal my process of learning about healing, as I focused more clearly on the nature of stage five. The first four stages had been about taking charge, regaining control of my body and my life. I was now firmly in control, it seemed—except for this wretched kidney bean. Perhaps stage five was something beyond control, beyond taking charge.

My little willingness had been growing over the last two years—willingness to consider the possibility of healing from a source beyond the visible, physical, and scientifically acceptable. During this trip I tried to suspend all doubt and gave myself a three-week time-out from resisting and challenging new beliefs that were ego-threatening.

I had absorbed the lessons of the *Course* to some degree in spite of my constant questioning and testing. In fact the small experiments I set up to test the concepts always gave me new evidence of the validity of the *Course's* upside-down ideas. Now for a space of three weeks I would be *willing* to allow the possibility that it was all true and only required my complete acceptance in order to be demonstrated. What did I have to lose?

For me, complete acceptance implied that I had a lot to lose. Complete acceptance meant yielding, giving over control and autonomy and even personality. How far could I go with acceptance? This would be my chance to find out.

What follows is a series of journal entries, recording the struggle I had with acceptance, and with what I thought it might require. The process of learning to accept, to surrender, was not a three-week task but had been under way for years, and these three weeks represented the final surge of intensity that made it possible for me to do it. Acceptance is accomplished in an instant, but it seemed that for me, months and years of internal struggle were necessary to get to that instant.

Our first morning on the road we were camped not far from home, near Mt. Hood. I had begun to keep a daily journal, writing in it every morning after meditating and walking.

August 26, 1985

Lesson 136:
"Sickness is a defense against the truth."

What a way to start a trip intended to heal the mind.

164

*I took a walk around the lovely Tollgate Camp-
ground, in the Mt. Hood National Forest. Sat on a rock
by the Sandy River. The words seeped slowly into my
soul and explained themselves. Often the meaning
doesn't come clear in meditation, but afterward, while
walking. The words "let," "allow" and "accept" were used
in this lesson. The lesson offers a prayer:*

"Sickness is a defense against the truth.
I will accept the truth of what I am,
And let my mind be wholly healed today."

*My mind be wholly healed. I keep forgetting. It's not
my body that needs healing, it's my mind. When I can
heal my thoughts my body will be well, as it always was.
I am not a body. Focusing on an imagined illness in my
body gives power to the belief that what I am, is: a body.*

*What I give my attention to becomes my God. When I
become my body I forget who/what I am: spirit. An expression of God, a part of God. I am as God created me,
whole, healthy, joy-filled. Spirit. My body is here for me
to use. It cannot feel pain or harbor sickness unless I
choose it. It can only die when I choose to die, when my
usefulness is over.*

"Let my mind be wholly healed today."

*The automatic protection given to my body by my
healed mind, says this lesson, must be preserved. If I let
my mind harbor attack thoughts (meaning I believe I can
be harmed, and therefore must defend myself), or yield to
judgment (meaning evaluating rightness or wrongness,
as if I could have a plan that is more right in its outcomes than God's), or make plans against uncertainties
to come (to protect myself) I have again identified my
Self with my body, and made my mind sick.*

165

Instant remedy from making my mind sick is to remember with clarity what must be healed, and tell myself:

"I have forgotten what I really am, for I mistook my body for myself. Sickness is a defense against the truth. But I am not a body. And my mind cannot attack. So I can not be sick."

Does it take effort? Or does it take allowing, accepting, and letting? Let it be. Stop the mind in its sick imaginings and let it be. Remember who/what I am. Give instant remedy for sick thoughts, attack thoughts, judgment, plan-making.

Plan-making. I know what that is. It's when my mind goes into a sort of mental fibrillation, dithering and blithering about the future—how will Jack fare as a widower again, what will my children do without me?

Sick, sick, sick. And that certainly isn't my body being sick, it's my mind. It plans what sort of surgery I will have next for this new tumor, what I will say to the doctors, how many days of classes I will miss Fall term, who will take over for me at work, and it speculates about what part of my body will fail next. Sick.

I will heal my mind, today, allow it to be healed, release it from these sick imaginings, and remember what I am. I am not a body, so none of these events will come to pass. No planning need be done.

Last night, we mused that there is a certain courage and dignity in not "getting religion" (foxhole religion, I think they call it) as the disease becomes more ominous. But I don't have that kind of mind, coping gamely with threatening and encroaching disease, accepting an early end like a trooper. I fight it and try to understand, to deal with it on a mental and spiritual basis.

This lesson says "accept." I am still fighting.

August 27, 1985: Steens Mountain in Southeast Oregon

Lesson 137:
"When I am healed I am not healed alone."

From this lesson: "Those who are healed become the instruments of healing." What does that mean? Write the book? Let it be known I'm available to help sick people? Visit hospitals? Apparently not: the Course *says I can not proselytize, but simply to ask for permission to gently help the sick person by my thoughts to see that his/her mind must be changed. Starting with myself.*

In this lesson, the words "...let yourself be healed ....let healing come ...let our minds be healed." How can I reconcile this with the effort I have put into taking charge of getting well and being in control of my life? It must be that there is, finally, a need for surrender.

August 28, 1985

Lesson138:
"Heaven is the decision I must make."

Decision. Choice. I can see the ego's world of pain and disaster. Or I can see heaven, which is right here, right now, but distorted and obscured by the ego's limiting belief system. It's as if I am in a room full of furniture and people and flowers and food and balloons, but with the light turned off. I am standing in the dark, unaware of the richness of the place where I am standing, and the party that is ready to begin when I turn on the light. It doesn't require sacrifice, just turning on the light and seeing what has been there all the time. All I give up is the absence of light, a nothing not a something.

August 29, 1985

Lesson 139:
"I will accept Atonement for myself."

*Atonement. I resisted that word when I first started
the* Course *because it smacked of sin, sacrifice and cru-
cifixion. But it means instead simply the undoing of the
ego and the healing of the belief in separation from God.
Some pronounce it at-one-ment. How I wish I could
finally and completely undo my stubborn ego. It hangs
on with increasingly ferocious determination. The closer
I get to waking up, the more frantic it becomes.*

August 30, 1985

Lesson 140:
"Only salvation can be said to cure."

*What a "coincidence" that the day we started on this
trip the lesson I was on in the Workbook was the first in
a series on sickness, healing, and cure.*

*I've finally started to do what the Workbook suggests:
spend one minute at each hour remembering the lesson
and asking for guidance. I set my watch to beep every
hour, then meditate for a minute or so. It's important—it
helps to keep the thing I'm working on simmering in my
unconscious, so that more and more insight is released.*

*In today's lesson, "Only salvation can be said to
cure," there's another of those words I resisted at first,
because of associations with early religious training. But
salvation is similar to atonement: we are saved from our
belief in the reality of separation, sin and guilt through
the change of mind that forgiveness and the miracle
bring.*

And a miracle is merely a change of mind that shifts our perception—from the ego's world of sin, guilt and fear to the higher Self's world of forgiveness.

I have to let go of my belief in sin and guilt, especially my own, before I can be permanently cured. Temporary healings from medical treatments, as I have experienced, will be only temporary because I still believe in sin, guilt, blame, judgment—and separation from God. Part of me believes that I have sinned and that I must earn God's love by punishing myself through sickness.

It's so hard to let go, to sacrifice all of these illusions I have created. I'm willing and ready to give up the illusion of sickness, but to do that apparently I have to give it all up. All my beliefs.

As Jack pointed out yesterday while we were walking, those illusions only appear to have served me well. I used judgment, planning, belief in goodness and badness, and belief in my body as who I am, to become professionally "rich and famous." And yet when I reached the pinnacle of rich-and-famous, ready to be launched yet higher into the stratosphere of power and worldly success, it all came apart—because of a power struggle in which I earnestly participated. The struggle, the conflict, the belief in how right I was, the determination to win, the belief that if I gave up or gave in I would lose, led to cancer.

Why have I had cancer three times? Why was I not cured last time? Why must I have it again? Maybe because I have not yet given up the illusions. I have read the message over and over that I resist the truth, that I resist giving up the illusion, and I have said to myself, "That doesn't mean me, because I have already changed my mind." But of course I haven't.

August 31, 1985

Lesson 141:
"My mind holds only what I think with God."

> [Note: Lessons 141-150 are review lessons, each starting
> with the single idea: "My mind holds only what I think
> with God," followed by a review of two earlier lessons.]

(Review of Lessons 121 and 122)
    121: "Forgiveness is the key to happiness."
    122: "Forgiveness offers everything I want."

Forgiveness offers everything *I want? Butter brickle
ice cream? Red shoes? Even freedom from this tumor?
Apparently it's not that direct or literal. We're talking
about what I* really *want: "peace, happiness, a quiet
mind, a certainty of purpose, and a sense of worth and
beauty that transcends the world."*

*Oh. And I was willing to settle for ice cream or new
shoes, and especially for getting rid of this tumor. But I
know from experience that getting rid of a tumor did not
automatically bring peace, happiness, or a quiet mind.*

The poetry of this lesson is lyrical:

> "Do you want care and safety, and the
> warmth of sure protection always? Do you want a
> quietness that cannot be disturbed, a gentleness
> that never can be hurt, a deep, abiding comfort,
> and a rest so perfect it can never be upset?
>
> All this forgiveness offers you, and more. It
> sparkles on your eyes as you awake, and gives
> you joy with which to meet the day. It soothes
> your forehead while you sleep, and rests upon
> your eyelids so you see no dreams of fear and
> evil, malice and attack. And when you wake

again, it offers you another day of happiness and peace. All this forgiveness offers you, and more."

Workbook, Lesson 122

What a huge reward for such a seemingly small effort. Simply forgive and be forgiven. The key to happiness.

o   o   o

I was beginning to face the unnegotiable need for forgiveness of everyone I believed had wronged me, even in small ways. Some people I would forgive again and again, melt the tip of the iceberg and find something new floating up a few days later. There was still a large iceberg submerged in my unconscious about Dr. Davidson, my first oncologist. My ego insisted he had tried to kill me.

To be healed, I must forgive everything. Everyone. I can't reserve out a person or event as special, too wrong to ever be forgiven. I had a dream, described in my journal:

September 1, 1985: Hagerman, Idaho

It is early, just after dawn. A dream :

I was going through old records. I came up with documents from my last operation, including a letter from Dr. Davidson describing that he had found not one but three tumors. One was a walnut-sized tumor in my foot. (Perhaps a flaw in my "under-standing?" Dreams often use puns to give a message.) *It was clear in the dream that either he had failed to send the tumors in for analysis or had failed to report the results to me. Hence, a third cancer would be his fault, right? Just as the second one was his fault.*

In the dream I collared nursing supervisors, directors, presidents, all those with any authority in this hospital, to tell them how I'd been damaged by this gross negligence. I wanted something done. But every time I began to tell my story of injury to someone, he or she would have to leave, having appointments, before I could even get to the part about how I'd been harmed. I would chase them down and insist on finishing my story, or find someone else to try to tell the whole story to.

I awoke suddenly, alert and feeling that this had been an important dream. So much was suddenly clear.

Yesterday I spent all day reflecting every hour on the day's lesson:

"My mind holds only what I think with God.
    Forgiveness is the key to happiness.
    Forgiveness offers everything I want."
                    Workbook, Lesson 141

I spent a lot of time doing little forgivenesses—closely monitoring my thoughts, banishing and correcting those thoughts that were not "thought with God." Feeling that now, finally, I was making progress, learning to forgive the moment I had a thought about some (usually imagined) wrong done to me. By monitoring my thoughts, I was able to see that most of the things I find to blame or judge someone for are my projection or my imagination.

I was beginning to feel hopeful that I would find what I seek. Peace of mind through union with God. Healing of the separation—union with all others, as well. Impossibility of anything in my life to forgive anyone for. I had accomplished all necessary forgiveness. Only the little daily cleaning-up stuff would continue. No more big ones.

Then the dream, the anger and frustration at trying to get someone to see and to agree that I had been harmed, to punish the bastard who had injured me so, to bring him before a tribunal.

So I haven't forgiven Dr. Davidson for causing my first cancer relapse. Haven't even started. In fact, it had to come in a dream because I had reserved out Dr. Davidson from forgiveness, since his sin was too great in my mind to be forgiven. The memory of that sin never came up during all my forgiveness exercises.

I've thought and said that Dr. Davidson did not cause my cancer relapse. I caused it myself, just as I caused my first cancer, by believing in sickness and by having a separated mind in need of healing. This awareness doesn't require guilt or blame but simple recognition, so that I can do something about it. But here it is—evidence that I have not forgiven him for the part he played. And until I do, I will not be healed.

Doing the lessons the way the Course *says I must has had an important effect. It brings up stuff from the unconscious and the barely conscious, repressed information, stuff I don't want to have to face. I don't want to have to forgive Dr. Davidson. I want him to be the villain in this piece, my* bete noir; *blaming him allows me to avoid taking complete responsibility for the sickness I have made, and gets me off the hook of having to do something about it.*

Then the guilt. I've been struggling with that, because the Course *says that guilt is responsible for sickness. What on earth could I feel guilty about, any more?*

Ken Wapnick's little book* has helped. It discusses where guilt comes from and why we all believe in sin and

---

* Wapnick, Ken, *Christian Psychology and A Course in Miracles*. Foundation for Inner Peace, Glen Ellen, CA *blame. It discusses projection, our favorite way to remove guilt from ourselves where it is too uncomfortable to bear, and put it out there on someone else instead. But we don't need to project if we can give up our belief in sin and judgment for everyone, including ourselves. Then we can let go of guilt, and let go of the need to project it by blaming someone else.*

Walking to the river this morning I saw that I had forgiven everyone I thought had injured me but had never directly addressed Dr. Davidson. I kept his wrong in reserve, set it aside from forgiveness, even repressed it as a need to forgive. I was willing to accept that sin does not exist, only error that can be corrected, and therefore doesn't even need forgiveness—except for that one, the really big one, the for-real sin that should never be forgiven, the sin Dr. Davidson committed against me.

What did he do? I meditated and did the exercise suggested in yesterday's lesson: reviewed every single one of his sins, not dwelling on any of them, just reviewing them. Asking myself, "Would I accuse myself of this?" And then recognizing his total innocence, knowing he did not intend to hurt me and in fact did not hurt me at all. If there was hurt, I did it to myself.

He was intent on having me in the control group for his research study, and didn't tell me I should have radiation, so I had a relapse...

...or did he tell me and I was too distraught to listen? And would I have chosen radiation, as afraid as I was of the deadly rays?

He didn't diagnose the relapse though I told him of a growing new lump six times in monthly visits...

...but since I didn't want to hear bad news did I perhaps not complain convincingly of my symptoms? Could he have been doing me a favor by not reinforcing my fears, since I was making myself sick by

174

believing in it and wanting him to recognize it and agree with me?

He didn't recommend chemotherapy after the relapse....

...why did I believe only chemotherapy could save me?

Carleen tells me Dr. Davidson was a pediatrician. He was so saddened by seeing children die of cancer that he changed specialties and became an oncologist and cancer researcher. When she told me this I didn't want to hear it, didn't want to have to think of him as a decent, kind, compassionate person who only wanted to heal and cure—who in fact wanted to find a cure for cancer through research—because I saw myself as victimized by his dedication to his research.

Dr. Davidson didn't cause my cancer and didn't cause my relapse. I was so afraid and so convinced that something was growing in my chest and that a relapse was imminent that I probably accelerated its growth through my intense fear and my passionate belief.

"Every thought is a prayer, and every prayer is answered."

I won't allow that to happen again but I'm aware that I could. I could turn a pimple into a virulent cancer with no seeming effort other than belief. My mind is that strong. And that's why it's so important that I use it only for good.

I will have what I seek. It will come, because I burn with desire for it. And the Course *tells me I will have it. Oneness with God, peace of mind, a healed mind. The body, maybe. It matters less now. Spiritual healing— healing of the mind—must come first, must come if nothing else comes.*

Just when I think I have reached a plateau where I might rest in my comfortable understanding and dare to *become complacent the next unsettling begins. And now in this unsettling I am aware for the first time of what the* Course *says is so: mighty companions * go with me from here on. There is a feeling of great underlying support holding me up and keeping me on the track.*

On the track. Before in my life I've always felt confused about the direction I was going, and was quick to jump on a new train passing by if it looked promising. Now I feel that I'm finally on the right train going in the right direction and need no longer be distracted by enticing side tracks, wondering if just maybe I should....

I know I will reach the place the train is going. I'm finally safe, guided, directed, kept from jumping the tracks. It's easier being on a train. Decision, evaluation and judgment are no longer needed.

September 4, 1985

Lesson 143:
"My mind holds only what I think with God."

(Review of Lessons 125 and 126)
   125: "In quiet I receive God's Word today."
   126: "All that I give is given to myself."

God's Word. Another resistance, to that phrase. The Course *uses those old conditioned-response words and phrases but redefines them. For meditation this lesson says today I should choose three times suitable for silence, and then*

---

* *A Course in Miracles Manual for Teachers,* page 10 (First edition)

"...give ten minutes set apart from listening to the world, and choose instead a gentle listening to the Word of God. He speaks from nearer than your heart to you. His Voice is closer than your hand. His Love is everything you are and that He is; the same as you, and you the same as He.

It is your voice to which you listen as He speaks to you... In quiet listen to your Self today, and let Him tell you God has never left His <Child>, and you have never left your Self."

Workbook, Lesson 125

Truth is not in any book. It is not in the Course. *It is within me. My inner voice will tell me the truth if I quiet my mind and listen for it. It can't be in any book, because the message is not always in words that can be clearly articulated and written down. Words cannot describe the truth. The* Course *has shown me the road to be on. But the truth comes in meditation, prayer, long walks alone, and in unexpected ways throughout the day. Sudden realizations and insights come from unlikely places and people and interactions.*

I read the lesson, meditate, and walk. Sometimes it feels as if nothing has happened. But later some fragment of understanding will come back to me from the lesson. All that is gained here is mine forever. I can never go back. And I cannot fail to find what I seek.

Here in the Grand Tetons heaven is now. Could I but keep this serenity and loveliness always. Of course I can if I choose.

Dinner last night was an extravaganza of fresh sun-ripened vegetables from the visit with our children (and their garden). We took a walk through the Park as the sun set. I wrote until after midnight while Jack practiced drawing. When we were both tired we made up only one of the beds so we could snuggle under all of the blankets and leave the windows open. Heat up the last cup of coffee for Jack, make a cup of cocoa for myself, settle down in bed with a book. Jack rubbed the typing tension out of my shoulders and we turned out the light very late.

This morning we were awake early as usual, refreshed in spite of little sleep. Jack made coffee and handed me a cup while I sat up in bed reading my morning lesson. He went for a walk. I meditated. We sat in the sun and shared some of our daughter's delectable homemade tomato juice and a huge cinnamon roll we picked up yesterday in Jackson. There are fresh peaches for later. Bliss.

After breakfast I walked to the lake to clarify what I didn't understood and deepen what is already clear. I found a quiet trail in the woods—it apparently goes all the way around Jackson Lake, quite a hike.

Bliss—writing in this home of ours on wheels, settled among the lodgepole pines, the aroma of fresh vegetable stew simmering for tonight, listening to a tape I bought in Jackson—two hours of the adagio movements from dozens of symphonies.

In Jackson we paid tribute to the Shopping God— something one is encouraged to do there. Shop and eat. We bought birthday presents for Jack's parents and found a Stetson cowboy hat for Jack, on sale for half price. Obviously he was meant to have it. Practiced restraint in restaurants—except for the raspberries in cream. Sweet cream and sour cream, sweetened, mixed and allowed to set, served in a parfait glass layered with raspberries.

This is what I fear I would have to do. Give this up, sacrifice the fun of the material world.

September 5, 1985: At the Continental Divide

Lesson 144:
"My mind holds only what I think with God."

(Review of Lessons 127 and 128)
    127: "There is no love but God's."
    128: "The world I see holds nothing that I want."

Jack and I have been talking about laws, since today's lesson suggests "No law the world obeys can help you grasp Love's meaning... Today we practice making free your mind of all the laws you think you must obey..." (Workbook, Lesson 127)

All day laws have been popping into my mind.

The Hiking Law: it must be at least six miles or it's not a hike, it's a walk. You must carry a day pack and a water bottle, and a Sierra cup on your belt. Maybe food. Little cans of juice. Half of the hike must be uphill, half downhill. Do not stop to rest too often, but you may stop every hour for five or ten minutes.

Jack says he has a Driving Law. If you accidentally pass up the place you planned to stop, do not go back. I remembered other Driving Laws: if someone in the car has to go to the bathroom but you don't, do not stop. If someone in the car is hungry but you aren't, do not stop. If someone in the car has to throw up, stop.

The Law of Tourism. Jack taught me about this one by revealing that it was a law and could be released. "I don't care if we don't do any sightseeing," he said. I felt guilty if we were in a place with sights to see and didn't see them. We usually forget to take the camera when there is a sight to see. The Law of Tourism says if there is something like Old Faithful of which hundreds of photographs have been published, you must nevertheless take your own picture of it.

179

So many laws. If attacked, defend yourself.

We have not taken full advantage of the magnificent scenery except to note it, sometimes to drink it in, mostly to use it as a backdrop for the inward journey.

We are leaving the Tetons behind today, heading north to Yellowstone two days earlier than planned. For both of us it was finished last night. It always hits us at the same time, the feeling of being finished with a vacation, needing to go home. The feeling is one of vague depression, restlessness, faint irritability, quietness. Then we look at each other and know it's time to go.

The motor home has been converted back into a vehicle. Yesterday it was home, with clutter everywhere, books piled on every surface, shoes and hiking boots and clothes tossed about, dinner simmering. Now everything is stowed, buttoned down, neat, businesslike, utilitarian. Jack turns the passenger seat around facing front again, and it is no longer a chair, but a navigator's seat.

Yesterday I wrote all morning while Jack drew. After lunch we headed out and walked six miles or so, part of the trail around the lake and back. I'm starting to let go of one piece of my past—that part that still feels deprived if I don't hike regularly. I needed to hike every weekend when I was thirty. My spiritual life was a shambles. Not believing in God any longer, hiking up an Oregon mountain trail was as close as I could ever get to Him. I don't need it in the same way now

Living on the edge of the woods on the farm there are many opportunities to get into the wilderness within moments of the front door. I haven't done enough of it because it wasn't hiking. According to my Law hiking had to be in the Cascades or the Wallowas or the Sierras—some granite mountain range.

Life since my hiking days has been at some level a longing for and a searching for the exhilaration and

180

glory I found on those mountain tops. The freedom and joy of scampering up mountain trails, surrounded by the saturated fragrance of sun-warmed pine needles, feeling the strength and power in my body, sitting on top of the world peeling the orange that was my reward for making it to the top. The freedom and exultation of running down the mountain creating a wind in my face.

This is where I belong. It is the right place, the right time. Hiking was fifteen years ago. Then, hiking represented release from all the assumptions and external laws that I believed governed me—traditional marriage, traditional motherhood, traditional religion. I began to make my own laws. Apparently hiking was one of them.

At the Continental Divide in Yellowstone Park we stopped and hiked (walked) two or three miles to Riddle Lake. A muscular wind was blowing, with just a few raindrops, and the tall skinny yellow pines swayed, rubbed together and squeaked eerily as we walked. The bright red WARNING!! sign at the trailhead told us there were bears and that they might attack, and if they did we should climb a tree or play dead. No problem!

I eyed the pines, little stubs of branches on the lower twenty feet of trunk, and knew I could shinny up one of these trees in seconds if I had to. Whenever we weren't talking, I yelled "No Bears!" just in case.

Metaphors leapt to mind as we walked. Pines in a high wind, resilient, bending and swaying to keep from breaking. "They must have a huge root system," I observed, "to bend so far without being uprooted." I was working on a cancer metaphor.

"No, look," Jack said. He pointed to a tree just in front of us on the trail, fallen with its entire root system revealed. There was no long tap root, no long side roots. Just a clump of dirt five feet across and maybe a foot deep, with a few tangled roots. So they do fall sometimes. Lots of times. Looking again, I see that the forest floor is

littered with downed pines, their inadequate root systems exposed.

Metaphors. After walking as far as we thought Riddle Lake was, all we could see was a large dried-up mudhole. Disgusted, I suggested we go back since the lake was obviously dried up this time of year. Jack insisted on continuing even though we could see no water ahead. We did continue, climbing a rise and around a ridge, and suddenly before us was a large mountain lake there on the top of the world, virtually on the Continental Divide at over 8000 feet—did one side of the lake drain into the Pacific and one side into the Atlantic? The water sparkled in the glimmers of sun peeking through the clouds. Water lilies floated around the edge. Across the lake a deer stooped to drink. We were the only humans up here on top of the world.

The lake was here the whole time I was contemplating the mudhole.

Nearly to Old Faithful, cars were stopped to watch buffalo graze. (Leaflet at the Park gate: WARNING! Fifteen people have been gored by buffalo in the Park this year! Buffalo can run thirty miles an hour while charging, which is three times as fast as you can run!)

Old Faithful performed on schedule, to an amphitheatre of hundreds of people. I wonder how many times in recorded history the phrase "Thar she blows!" has been repeated here. Viewing such a sight turns on the shopping gene, it seems, because most of the hundreds of people left the geyser after it had erupted and followed us straight to the gift shop.

Indian stuff, pots, beads, cups, camping stuff, jewelry, ice cream, popcorn, big log burning in the fireplace—it's chilly enough today that a wood fire feels good. Buffalo horns! Big mounted buffalo horns. I wanted to buy a set, to mount on the front of the R.V.

"WARNING!! Twenty-three people have been gored by R.V.s in the Park this year. R.V.s can run sixty miles an hour, which is six times as fast..." We didn't buy the horns. Jack turns off his shopping gene the minute he sees the word souvenir on the sign.

The bubbling "paint pots" were extravagant—boiling mud, boiling water, geysers erupting and the brisk wind blowing the steam straight out along the ground, trees dead and white for two feet up the trunk. Acrid sulphur smell.

September 6, 1985

Lesson 145:
"My mind holds only what I think with God."

(Review of Lessons 129 and 130)
    129: "Beyond this world there is a world I want."
    130: "It is impossible to see two worlds."

I read ahead in the lessons last night, wanting to see "how it comes out." Scared myself. It comes out that I will devote my life to being available to those who need my help, my light, my teaching. Give up the world I have and become a missionary?

When we woke up I rolled over and asked Jack, "What if the cost of getting well is that I have to hang out a shingle, 'Miracle Worker. Inquire Within.'" His answer: "If you still call it 'cost,' then you haven't understood what you read last night."

In his voice, there was a "But..." which I pursued. It turned out to be, he doesn't want me to give up the world I have and become a missionary. (Afraid giving up the world I have includes him? That's what I'm afraid of.)

This morning the answer was there in the review lesson:

"Beyond this world there is a world I want."
"It is impossible to see two worlds."
Workbook, Lesson 145

In meditation, I asked for clarification about giving up the world. This was the comforting message:

"The world is a 'negative,' like a white-on-black photographic image. You don't have to leave it or change it. Just stay where you are and reverse the image to reality. You cannot see two worlds at the same time.

Behind this world is heaven—the richness of the world with the lights turned on. It is impossible to see the world of the ego and at the same time the world *without* the limitations and belief structure of the ego. And vice versa."

o   o   o

I asked for more. It was this:

"Dear child, do not be afraid.
You are well.
You always have been
and you always will be.
You are not a body.
You are free."

Butte, Montana
Butte is a city built by copper mines, the big ugly open pit looming over everything. The mine is closed

now, and Butte has quietly gone to seed. It needs a miracle, rejuvenation. But it's a comfortably shabby old western town without a gaudy facade.

Walking down the street I tripped twice on the broken-up sidewalk, would have fallen if Jack hadn't been holding my arm. Once I was staring down at the sidewalk and still tripped over it. Jack said he'd urge me to sue the city for my injuries, except in court they would probably ask him if I was clumsy and he'd either have to perjure himself or I'd lose the case.

September 7, 1985: Couer d'Alene, Idaho

Lesson 146:
"My mind holds only what I think with God."

(Review of Lessons 131 and 132)
131: "No one can fail who seeks to reach the truth."
    132: "I loose the world from all I thought it was."

I haven't failed because of this new kidney bean. Nor will I. Lesson 131 speaks of looking for permanence, love, safety, immortality—worthy goals—but guaranteed to end in failure while we look "...for permanence in the impermanent, for love where there is none, for safety in the midst of danger; immortality within the darkness of the dream of death." (Workbook, Lesson 131)

> *Lesson 132 continues:*
> "I loose the world from all I thought it was."
> "...there is no world apart from what you wish ...change but your mind on what you want to see, and all the world must change accordingly ...you made the world you see ..."

"...the world does not exist. And if it is indeed your own imagining, then you can loose it from all things you ever thought it was by merely changing all the thoughts that gave it these appearances. The sick are healed as you let go all thoughts of sickness..."

"You are as God created you."

All of that means, must mean, that I am created in God's image and therefore limitless, immortal, and perfect. I know the power of the mind to create sickness and have in the past felt at the mercy of my powerful mind which seemingly operated on its own, busily creating cancers. But God is in my mind. My higher mind. I have allowed my ego to create sickness, to seek meaningless goals, and to seek worthy goals but in all the wrong places.

September 8, 1985: Couer d'Alene

Lesson 147: "My mind holds only what I think with God."

(Review of Lessons 133 and 134)
    133: "I will not value what is valueless."
    134: "Let me perceive forgiveness as it is."

Value what is valueless. What could that be?

We are staying in an R.V. park a few blocks from the lake. We walked for a couple of hours last night along Lakeshore Drive to a lovely causeway across one end of the lake, in front of the posh North Shore Hotel, where the rich or envious gather to play. Any one of the hundreds of boats in the marina could have bought our whole farm. It's of interest, but not appealing. Maybe at some time in the past it would have been. Maybe we would have felt envy. We don't. It's only of interest. How could anything be better than what we have? Life is utterly complete, lacking nothing. We are valuing what is valuable.

Reviewing lesson 131 again this morning, the lines that stood out had to do with sacrifice:

"Everything you seek but <Heaven> will fall away. Yet not because it has been taken from you. It will go because you do not want it." (Workbook, Lesson 131)

Later, flipping through the book, this :

"I am not asked to make a sacrifice
To find the mercy and the peace of God.
...The mercy and the peace of God are free.
Salvation has no cost.
It is a gift that must be freely given and received."

Workbook, Lesson 343

September 9, 1985

Lesson 148: "My mind holds only what I think with God."

(Review of Lessons 135 and 136)
    135: "If I defend myself I am attacked."
    136: "Sickness is a defense against the truth."

What on earth can this mean, a "defense against the truth?"

It was here, reading this lesson the first time, that I first realized how little of the message of the Course *I was really accepting. I understand it intellectually, have witnessed the power of the mind to create sickness or health. I have on occasion even experienced the holy instant it speaks of, those moments when I am wholly aware of and know the truth of my oneness with God. When I am totally in my higher mind.*

Yet here were the paragraphs from Lesson 136 which left me confused and a little panicky as I began to comprehend what it was really saying:

"Sickness is a decision. It is not a thing that happens to you, quite unsought, which makes you weak and brings you suffering. It is a choice you make, a plan you lay, when for an instant truth arises in your own deluded mind, and all your world totters and prepares to fall. Now are you sick, that truth may go away and threaten your establishments no more.

How do you think that sickness can succeed in shielding you from truth? Because it proves the body is not separate from you, and so you must be separate from the truth. You suffer pain because the body does, and in this pain are you made one with it. Thus is your true identity preserved, and the strange, haunting thought that you might be something beyond this little pile of dust silenced and stilled. For see, this dust can make you suffer, twist your limbs and stop your heart, commanding you to die and cease to be."

I can accept that I created my own sickness, and I thought I knew the reasons. The first time, it was the irresolvable conflict and strife in my Alaska job and in my marriage. I left Alaska, and finally the marriage. The second time, it was the stress and tension of my job. I gave that up for a lower-stress job.

Haven't I finally gotten it right? Marriage to an angel who was obviously sent to care for me, interesting job, in control of my time, living on a peaceful farm and daily seeking to know the truth. All the things that conspired to help me create a cancer as a way out before are gone from my life. I have nothing to escape from now.

> "...it is a choice you make, a plan you lay, when for an instant truth arises in your own deluded mind, and all your world totters and prepares to fall. Now are you sick, that truth may go away..."
>
> *Workbook, Lesson 136*

I am creating sickness to avoid the truth? To avoid knowing, truly, my oneness with God? But that is all I want. How could it threaten me?

Slowly, slowly, meditating and walking in the wilderness quiet, I begin to see. It threatens me because of what I believe I will have to give up. Sacrifice. Also an illusion, but a powerful one.

Sacrifice. What might I have to give up? Only the fun of being critical of others, sarcasm, the sharp needle of judgment, gossip. The self-indulgence of feeling injured, the thrill of attack and of marshalling my resources for defense. Planning for unknown eventualities. Staying in control. Especially staying in control. Believing in all of this delusionary world I have made, believing that it is better, stronger, and more successful than God's world, His plan.

I am afraid to let go.

The lesson goes on with a meditation: "...I will accept the truth of what I am, and let my mind be wholly healed today."

In Goodbye to Guilt, *Jerry Jampolsky speaks of the necessity for the mind to be healed, wholly healed, before the body can be wholly healed. What is healing of the mind? Lesson 136 says:*

189

"Healing will flash across your open mind, as peace and truth arise to take the place of war and vain imaginings... Now is the body healed, because the source of sickness has been opened to relief...this removes the limits you had placed upon the body by the purposes you gave to it. As these are laid aside, the strength the body has will always be enough to serve all truly useful purposes. The body's health is fully guaranteed, because it is not limited by time, by weather or fatigue, by food and drink, or any laws you made it serve before. You need do nothing now to make it well, for sickness has become impossible."

Hey! It's not asking me to do fifteen minutes a day of aerobic exercise, refuse red meat, take megavitamins, or jog till I drop. In fact, it says "it [the body] is not limited by food or drink, or any laws you made it serve before." This could be less threatening than I imagined.

If I am truly one with God and with my fellows what will that mean? No more kvetching, no competition, no laying plans for success. No enemies. No more blaming others for my problems. No more anger. Not even righteous anger. Only love. Can I give it all up? Now I see the truth of the phrase, "...all your world appears to totter and prepare to fall," from Lesson 136.

It feels like I'm giving up my true self, my personality. In fact, though, it is reclaiming my truest, highest Self which has been there all the time, waiting for me to wake up from the dream. What will my friends think?

My closest friend has already said to me, "I liked your lower self better."

My lower self (my ego) relished our long lunches together, self-indulgent immersions in negativity and judgment. Giggling at our perception and wit in being critical of others. Over the past two years my delight in such activities has faded, my discomfort growing until it has become painful to participate. Our long friendship is being tested. It must change or be put aside.

Jack's observation about laws we made applies again here: my ego-techniques were reinforced and verified as effective by the payoff of status, prestige, salary, and respect. That's what I'm reluctant to sacrifice.

I thought about that. Is it true? Has my ego brought me all that I want? No. It has brought me burnout from the stress. It brought me frustration and disappointment, particularly when I was unwilling to give up control. It brought me two failed marriages. It brought me the illusion of a limited "fame and fortune," all of which turned to ashes when cancer came.

I recognize my deep and powerful resistance to accepting the truth of what I am and letting my mind be wholly healed. I understand the urgency of it, yet, I resist. My ego is waging its last desperate battle and God waits quietly, knowing I will find what I seek.

"No one can fail who seeks to reach the truth."
Workbook, Lesson 131

I will find what I seek.

Tuesday, September 10, 1985: Coming Home

On the way home. Anxious to leave after visiting our children in Cheney. Jack's parents arrived with zucchini as we were getting ready, then called as soon as they got home again to say they forgot to put in the tomatoes. We went by and got the tomatoes. Posed for a picture. Every cell in my body wanted to be headed for home.

Picked up the dogs at Barbara's. They were delighted to see us, and had obviously been well-loved and well-

cared-for while we were gone. They were brushed out and happy. Joplin was so excited to see us she jumped up on my lap in the motor home, and while Jack was paying for their care she leaped against the door, pushed it open, and tumbled right out on the road. Just picked herself up and chased around merrily, so happy to be out and headed home.

As we rounded the last curve before the farm, Fishhawk Creek flashed a welcome, splashing over stones in its tunnel of alder trees. I remembered the hot August day we had first received that cool welcome, wondering then how much farther it was to the farm the realtor was taking us to see.

In the September twilight we turned into the driveway, let the excited dogs out of the motor home, and just sat, soaking in the peace, the lamp in the window, the fragile velvet mist drifting over the pasture. Wispy fog had appeared ten miles earlier as we passed through the tiny town of Mist—named for the morning and evening ground fog so predictable this time of year.

The honeysuckle draping the back porch scented the air with lush fragrance. We could hear the creek a few yards away as we carried things into the house. The garden had taken advantage of our absence to fill itself with weeds—blackheart, my nemesis. One year I pulled every blackheart from the patch of ground by the road, before they could develop their pretty pink seedheads, and planted meadow flowers there instead. It was still clear of blackheart. I would have to tackle the garden next. Maybe next year.

The house was clean and quiet, and cold. Three weeks' worth of mail, including two dozen catalogs, covered the big round oak table in the kitchen. A bottle of wine stood on the table, and a note from a friend who had come out and stayed four days, alone with herself for

*the first time in her life. "There's a lot of warmth here,"
she wrote. "It must come from you both."*

*Jack crumpled mailbox flyers to start a fire in the
woodstove. Grumbling, he went out the back door to chop
wood— the woodbox was empty.*

*I stepped out onto the front porch to see how the
flowers had fared. The red fuschia was ablaze, enjoying
this cool damp weather. The pink one looked tired and
listless. Scarlet petunias and yellow marigolds had
spread to fill the flower bed, and pink and purple asters
were so tall they were leaning on each other.*

*With the fire crackling and warming the corners of
the great room, we sorted the mail. The day we left on
this trip, I had ordered new checkbooks, and here they
were. Four boxes. I had paused for long minutes while
filling out the order form. 150? 300? 600? The first 300
checks had lasted nearly two years. No telling what the
future would bring—maybe 150 would be plenty. No. I
had checked the 600 box decisively.*

*We heated some soup and made toast. Started a pot
of coffee. Checked the refrigerator and made a grocery
list. Unwrapped a box of tulip bulbs, eight each of white,
apricot, light red, dark red, flaming yellow, purple, and
a new near-black. I would have to plant these before the
faculty was to report back on Monday, five days from
now. Already the pace was quickening. There was a letter
from the Dean, laying out the schedule for the first two
weeks, meetings and advising and planning sessions.
Not much time in there to prepare for the new classes I
was scheduled to teach. But first, Thursday and Friday,
the doctor appointments. Just one more day.*

*I poured myself a cup of coffee and took a new
magazine into the bathroom where the claw-footed tub
was filling. This issue had healing meditations for each
day of October, and an article on how to use the power of
thought. And another on "the wellspring of Life and*

Perfection at the center of your being upon which you may draw." This is how I would end the trip. The healing trip.

Wednesday, September 11, 1985

I've spent this day, this one precious day, doing exactly what I wished to do, before the appointment with the surgeon tomorrow and the oncologist the next day. I wasn't prepared for the phone call at four o'clock. I had ground wheat, made three loaves of whole wheat bread and two large loaves of Jack's favorite golden raisin bread. Pulled the refrigerator out from the wall and scrubbed it while it's still relatively empty. Got some letters ready to mail. Then the phone call. It was Dr. Michael's appointment desk.

"Doctor says you already know about this: he wants to do a little biopsy on your chest. He can do it right here in the clinic. He'll do it Monday at two o'clock."

"But..." I protested, "I had an appointment to see him tomorrow at two-thirty..."

"Oh, no," she explained. "He'll be in Boston tomorrow. I just heard him tell the nurse he won't be here, but he said he wanted to do your biopsy right away."

She said soothing words about what a simple procedure this was to be, done right in the clinic, no problem.

This was bollixing my careful, fragile plans. I made a last attempt. "I would like to talk to him before he schedules a biopsy. I don't think the tumor has grown, and would like to give it some more time before a biopsy."

"Oh, well, of course, he'll see you first, and if you do decide to go ahead with the biopsy he can just do it right then," she replied.

194

I hung up. Tomorrow was off. Another day of reprieve. Why was I so reluctant to have a simple procedure? Not wanting to know the "truth?" Not wanting to disturb that delicate, healing area? Or, more likely: not wanting to climb back on the carousel, subject myself to the intense pressure of the beliefs of medical science. Not wanting my building and growing truth and understanding to be threatened by exposure to that illusory world with its relentless belief system.

Talking to Jack, who hurts having to think about this, we devised a plan. I will go ahead and see Dr. Paul on Friday as scheduled. He is not a surgeon, he won't insist on cutting. If the diagnosis from Dr. Paul is a happy one, I'll see the radiation oncologist in a month to verify and confirm. If the lump has grown I'll agree to have a mammogram, and any other non-invasive tests that might yield a diagnosis. Then we'll wait a month, and do the tests again. Then reconsider, decide what to do next. But I will decide only after intensive meditation and asking the Holy Spirit to guide me, to tell me the right path to take.

We talked some more. What is it that we both resist so much in submitting to a doctor? Maybe it's that we've both had evidence that doctors can make a person sick as readily as they can make him well; that medicine can even kill rather than cure. Why then should it also be hard to accept that our own curative powers are more certain, more gentle, more permanent? Medical science has certainly offered us less.

At times I feel a tug, a wanting to just give in, to give up, to go along with the program. Go to the doctor, have the tests, have the biopsy, accept their beliefs in place of my own, have more surgery, have the last-chance chemotherapy that would make me sick, make me bald, and damage my heart. Accept their prognoses, and die.

*Make them happy. Confirm their beliefs. Satisfy their
need to be right about me.*

*Why would I have such insane inclinations? Jack
says it's sheer perversity, and he read to me a story from
a magazine:*

*"When I was 12, my best friend and I broke a window
playing baseball. We looked around to see if anyone had
seen us. No one was in sight except my younger brother.
We went over and offered him a piece of candy not to tell.
He refused it.*

'I'll give you my baseball,' I said.

'No.'

*'Then what about MY baseball and my new glove?' my
friend added.*

'No!'

'Well, what do you want?'

'I wanna tell.'"

*Why should this perverse wish sometimes surface, in
spite of the gifts of peace and healing being offered to me
by the Holy Spirit now? Would it give my ego some
twisted pleasure to climb on the carousel and go through
the usual, the predicted, the expected, and to die on
schedule? That is so upside down that I can't believe it is
still in my mind but apparently on rare occasions it is.
The good news is, it happens now only in flashes and is
overpowered by the growing understanding of how true
healing really takes place.*

*And why does it bother me that anyone who knows
about the path I want to take will think I'm crazy? Marie
called a few weeks ago, Marie from the summer writing
workshop. Marie is writing a book about her breast
cancer. She chattered and babbled happily on for about
half an hour, when for some dumb reason I decided to
tell her that my book was changing because a new lump*

had been found in my breast. I told her how I intended to deal with it, essentially by refusing to accept the beliefs of the doctors and by knowing I was well. Her voice changed, grew tentative and distant. "Well, I hope you're right," she said, then realized she must be keeping me and rang off.

I can't think of anyone, except my mother and Jack, with whom I can discuss this. No one who would understand and encourage me, and not say, "Well, I hope you're right." I remember those times in the past when I've read of a Christian Scientist who succumbed to cancer after refusing treatment, and have shaken my head at the ignorance and belief in "magic" that represented.

I told Jack, while stirring the chili for dinner, that I felt I was on the right track. I told him the most important thing was to heal my mind even if it meant I would die with an unhealed body. He did not agree, couldn't agree, couldn't speak, just shook his head and swallowed hard. I added that to be physically well and spiritually sick would be worse than to die with a healed mind. He's working on that. But tonight he fell asleep at eight o'clock, head on my shoulder on the couch. He wants to escape.

Thursday, September 12, 1985

Today was awful. Jack was clearly depressed, hasn't shaved for three days, upset stomach, grumpy and quiet. Fell asleep in a chair right after lunch and slept all afternoon. Escaped. Maybe it's important that I not share my occasional doubts and fears with him and especially that I not talk, even in hypothetical terms at this point, about dying.

I need for him to be able to continue to be positive and certain, or at least to pretend to be. And why should I share any negative thoughts with him? It only reinforces them for me and stimulates his own fears. He reminded me today that he had already lost one loved one, and is not inclined to be totally objective when I talk about dying—even dying with a healed mind. Easy for me to say—I'm in control here. He only gets to watch helplessly as I make my decisions.

Tomorrow the oncologist. Then there will be no retreat, we'll be into it. Just felt of the kidney bean. It seems to me to be a hard, marble-sized lump, with little "fingers" that reach up under the nipple.

This morning when I woke and felt the lump and there it was, hard and fixed, Jack caught me in the act. He protested, asking why I insist on thinking of it as real, telling me to just quit feeling of it. "How would you behave," I shot back, "if you had had testicular cancer twice and now there were new hard lumps in your testicles? Would you serenely believe them not to be there and just go on with your life, and never feel of them?" No answer. He can't say. It hasn't happened to him.

When I had the chest wall cancer I felt of it every night, then didn't sleep. Every night for six months. Mornings, too. Couldn't stop myself.

Every time I've been certain I had cancer, doctors have repeatedly assured me I did not. "It's probably a cyst." "It's your imagination." "It's your rib." "It's probably a benign chondrosarcoma." "It's your imagination."

Now that I feel certain I do not have cancer, doctors have tried to convince me I am probably wrong. So tomorrow I have to remember that. If Dr. Paul seems certain it's malignant that should reassure me. Since this time I don't feel that I am sick.

Chapter Six

The Fifth Stage:
Acceptance

*F*riday, September 13, 1985 was my daughter Kelley's twenty-fifth birthday. I woke anxious and hyperactive. It was on Laurie's birthday that the second cancer was confirmed.

The lump was still there. The movie was still running. I tried to meditate. During meditation, I had a clear vision of Dr. Paul stepping back from the examination table and saying, "There's nothing there." I tried to calm myself with this vision, but was still jumpy. The appointment was in the afternoon, and I had to get centered, somehow. I got up and put on my jeans to go hiking.

The hills above our house are criss-crossed with abandoned logging roads, offering endless combinations of solitary excursions and explorations. Today I walked fast, always heading uphill. I was angry at God, feeling betrayed again that I had spent these weeks learning to heal, and was not healed. What had gone wrong? What hadn't I done? I began to ask my questions aloud, passionately challenging, daring God to answer me.

"Why haven't I been healed? Haven't I forgiven everyone and myself?" I demanded.

No answer.

Again. "Haven't I given up judgment, and attack, and defenses?"

No answer.

"Haven't I accepted Your will?"

I was burning with intensity, churning up the hill and hurling challenges at God.

"Haven't I accepted Your will?" I shouted.

Now I became aware of a Presence in front of me on the road, not visible, but certainly palpable. This Presence seemed to be moving at the same rate I was walking, staying just in front of me. I heard a quiet response:

"Have you?"

Good. We were truly going to engage this question.

"Of *course* I have. I *have* accepted Your will." I insisted.

"Have you really?" asked the Presence.

"Of course," I said.

"Oh," the Presence said.

I walked on, considering this response. I had worked hard to give up planning, to accept God's will for me. "God's will for me is perfect happiness," according to the *Course.* If that were true, why not accept God's will? I obviously had not accomplished perfect happiness with my own will. I renewed the argument.

"Yes, I certainly have accepted Your will."

"Have you really?" asked the Presence.

"Yes, damn it!" I insisted.

"Oh."

I considered this—angry, defiant, rebellious at this persistent response. Another mile passed, and the Presence still walked with me, silent.

I tried again.

"I *have* accepted Your will."

This time I heard:

"Would you accept my will if my will is that you die young?"

"Of course not!" I was stunned. "What do you think all of this has been about? Of course I wouldn't accept that!"

No response.

This was crazy. Why would I go through all that I had been through only to give up in the end to "God's will" that I die? How could God will that I die? God's will for me was perfect happiness. I could never accept dying as God's will. Why had He asked such a stupid question?

"Why would you ask such a stupid question?" I raged. "Of *course* I wouldn't accept Your will if it meant that I would die."

No response.

Could it be that there were some things I didn't understand yet, about dying? Maybe dying with a healed mind *was* perfect happiness. But if I truly accepted God's will even if it meant that I would die, then I *would* die. All of this work, all of the stages of getting well, would have been for nothing.

Well, maybe not for nothing. I'm well on the way to a healed mind. Why is dying such a big deal, anyway? Maybe I've become obsessed with that one issue, overlooking the reality that dying only means moving on to the next plane, giving up the body with all its limitations and its temptations to ignore and distort the truth. Would it really be so awful to accept that I will die? I will in any case, so what's the difference whether it's now or later?

I walked for miles, struggling, that question shimmering in the air. "Would you accept my will if my will is that you die young?"

Would I?

I had not accepted God's will if I had reserved out this one eventuality. It was like reserving out Dr. Davidson from forgiveness. If I had reservations about anyone, I had not accomplished true forgiveness. If I had reservations about accepting God's will in this one instance, I had not accepted it at all. All or nothing. Complete submission.

Complete submission, apparently, was nearly impossible for me. I was finally willing to give over almost everything, but total surrender was out of the question. Was it really necessary? Did I have to do it?

Apparently I did. The Presence was gentle but unyielding. All or nothing.

I gave up. What did I have to lose? It appeared that I would die young in any case, so what difference did it make? I surrendered. I would accept God's will for me, even if it meant I would die.

Something large and heavy shifted inside me, lightened and took wings. I didn't have to announce this decision. It seemed to be known and accepted by this Presence. The emotions overwhelming me were unexpected and indescribable—not resignation, but freedom. Not anguish but joy. Not anxiety but peace. I was surrounded by love.

o   o   o

We drove to the clinic in silence. I had told Jack about my vision of Dr. Paul during morning meditation, but I found it impossible to tell him yet what had happened on the hike or how I felt now. He seemed to have lost his depression, however, and had regained his quiet confidence.

Dr. Paul's examination was efficient but careful and thorough. He had been briefed by Dr. Roberts and Dr. Michaels about the kidney bean, and he expected to find it larger after this month of inattention. He asked me to sit up, then to lie down. Finally he stepped back from the table and his usually impassive face registered puzzlement.

"There's nothing there," he said.

And there was nothing there.

Dr. Paul shook my hand, ignoring the tears in my eyes, and sent me on my way.

I danced out into the waiting room trying not be be too unseemly in my delight, and found Jack asleep in his chair. I shook him awake. My eyes shining, I asked him how he could sleep at a time like this!

"It's easy," Jack responded. "I knew how it would come out."

o   o   o

The final stage, the fifth stage in getting well, is acceptance. Not acceptance of an early death but acceptance of God's will, which is perfect happiness. I had not understood what that final stage was until I recognized the need for complete surrender. After all the taking charge, being in control, and managing my own recovery, it was necessary finally to give up control and to surrender to healing. Allow, let, accept the healing that I had struggled so hard to have.

"Whoever clings to this life shall lose it, and whoever loses his life shall save it."

Luke 17:33

o   o   o

"What could have happened to it?" I asked Dr. Roberts a month later. He had just confirmed that there was no longer a lump in my breast.

"Well," he pondered, "it could have been a cyst."

"Hard and immovable?" I prodded him with his own words. Hard and immovable usually meant cancer, he had reminded me when he wanted me to begin treatment immediately.

"Well, then it might have been scar tissue," he responded.

"Does scar tissue go away? Overnight?" I asked.

"Well, no. Of course not." He was getting testy.

"What could it have been, then?" I asked.

"I don't know what it was. I just don't know. I just don't know," he said. He clearly wanted to drop the subject, so I let him off the hook.

More than seven years later Dr. Roberts finally uses the C word with me: Cure. He still doesn't understand it, but he shares my joy, and celebrates my continued wellness. So do Dr. Paul and Dr. Michaels. They have participated in true healing and they are delighted.

God's will for me is perfect happiness. Now I understand the final stage of healing.

"And every miracle is possible the instant that the Son of God perceives his wishes and the Will of God are one."

A Course in Miracles, Text
p. 516 (first edition)

Chapter Seven

Post-~~Mortem~~ Miracle

September, 1992

"*W*hat would you do if you got sick again?"
Several have asked me that question out loud
and it hangs in the air unspoken by others. I have
given it some thought. At first I was confident I
would go for a repeat performance, secure now in
my trust in God, and without trust in medicine.

Now, I don't know.

Not even knowing for sure about myself, I
could not recommend a course of action for
anyone else. This book is not a recommendation

for a course of action, nor is it a blueprint. It is a personal story, intended to give hope, encouragement, and support to those with a similar challenge.

What would I do if I got sick again?

Knowing the source of my wholeness, I would not make such an important decision alone. I would pray for guidance and hope to understand God's Will for me, which is perfect happiness. His Will might include turning to traditional medicine for help, giving concrete form to my intention to heal. It might also include non-traditional forms. It would surely include seeking to heal my mind of its belief that I am a body and can be sick.

I have no doubt that traditional medical treatment was an essential part of my recovery from cancer—fortunately, I complemented medical treatment with spiritual healing. Learning to heal my mind, however, took as long as the treatments. Had I chosen to abandon physical approaches back then, it would have placed a terrible burden on a mind yet untrained and unhealed.

Surgery removed the obvious physical symptom, the tumor, making it easier to focus on my wholeness. Radiation and chemotherapy gave my unhealed mind the assurance that I was doing something, something in which many experts placed their trust. Medicine gave me time to learn the true source of healing. Choosing traditional therapy gave tangible form to my intention to heal, and gave me the comfort and security of the known while I explored the unknown.

While we live in the world of perception—the world *A Course in Miracles* calls the dream—we see the body as concrete reality, and it responds to concrete methods. The *Course* suggests that illness sometimes has a sufficiently strong hold over the mind to render a person temporarily unable to accept Divine help in healing. At such times, it goes on, it is safer to rely temporarily on physical healing devices. The sick are already in a fear-weakened state, or they would not be sick. Anything that increases fear, including "premature exposure to a miracle," should not be used.*

What would I do if I got sick again?

I would ask for Divine help in healing my mind that thought it could be sick and separate from God and others. I would go within to acknowledge any fear, guilt or lack of forgiveness that might have left me open to sickness, and would ask for help in correcting those mistakes. I would ask for guidance about medical treatments that might be recommended.

Finally, I would surrender completely to God's Will for me, recognizing that His Will is only my happiness.

Does this mean I might die? It means that at some point I will choose to discard my body when its usefulness is done. It need not be through sickness. I will ask for guidance even about that: have I fulfilled my function here? This is different from the death wish, the ego's goal of death. It is described lyrically in *The Song of Prayer*:

"Yet there is a kind of seeming death that has a different source. It does not come because of hurtful thoughts and raging anger at the universe. It merely signifies the end has come for usefulness of body functioning. And so it is discarded as a

---

* *A Course in Miracles, Text,* page 20 (First edition)

choice, as one lays by a garment now outworn.

This is what death should be; a quiet choice, made joyfully and with a sense of peace, because the body has been kindly used to help the Son of God along the way he goes to God. We thank the body, then, for all the service it has given us...

We call it death, but it is liberty. It does not come in forms that seem to be thrust down in pain upon unwilling flesh, but as a gentle welcome to release. If there has been true healing, this can be the form in which death comes when it is time to rest a while from labor gladly done and gladly ended. Now we go in peace to freer air and gentler climate, where it is not hard to see the gifts we gave were saved for us. For Christ is clearer now; His vision more sustained in us; His Voice, the Word of God, more certainly our own.

This gentle passage to a higher prayer, a kind forgiveness of the ways of earth, can only be received with thankfulness. Yet first true healing must have come to bless the mind with loving pardon for the sins it dreamed about and laid upon the world. Now are its dreams dispelled in quiet rest. Now its forgiveness comes to heal the world and it is ready to depart in peace, the journey over and the lessons learned."*

---

* *The Song of Prayer: Prayer, Forgiveness, Healing,* page 16.
Foundation for Inner Peace, Glen Ellen, CA

After Life

When I recall what life was like before I got sick and got well, it is a dream—often a nightmare—faintly remembered. Now that I am "weller than well" life is an experience to be savored, joy and peace largely having replaced fear and anger.

I am still learning. I didn't finish the *Course* until a year or so after my personal miracle, and I am still studying it. I still have occasional health problems which I would call minor, except for the *Course's* suggestion that there is no order of difficulty in illusion, or in miracles. If a wart on my finger ignited in me the same passion to understand as did cancer, I would seek a miracle of healing for the wart. But it doesn't, so I let it go.

The greatest miracle of all is the one promised in the *Workbook*, Lesson 137:

> *"And as you let yourself be healed you see all those around you, or who cross your mind, or whom you touch or those who seem to have no contact with you, healed along with you. Perhaps you will not recognize them all, nor realize how great your offering to all the world, when you let healing come to you. But you are never healed alone. And legions upon legions will receive the gift that you receive when you are healed."*

This book is part of the extension of that miracle. I have been healed. As I have let myself be healed, you are healed along with me. And as you are healed, so will we all be healed along with you.

We are one mind, connected through the Mind of God, holy, whole and innocent. Healed.

Annotated Bibliography

The Art of Healing Prayer. Unity School of Christianity. An eight-page pamphlet outlining the steps in praying for healing.

Augsberger, David, *The Freedom of Forgiveness: Seventy Times Seven*. The Moody Bible Institute of Chicago, 1970.

Brand, Dr. Paul and Yancey, Philip, *Healing*. Multnomah Press, Portland, Oregon, 1984. An interesting discussion of what is operating at the physical level in what appears to be a metaphysical healing. The author is a physician who does not believe in "miracles" in the supernatural sense. He knows of many who have participated in healing services, have been prayed for, and sometimes healed, but not in ways that counteracted the laws governing anatomy. He defines "divine healing" as a supernatural intervention that reverses natural laws governing our bodies, and find it to be very rare indeed.[*]

---

[*]...rare, but not unknown. If such a reversal of "natural laws" occurred even once, it constitutes evidence that what we regard as natural laws may be at least partly maintained by the immense power of our collective belief in such laws. If we could believe that restoration of a missing eye or leg, or the cure of an incurable disease, was as simple and as probable as supernatural healing of a wart, such healings would perhaps occur on a regular basis. Recent evidence that this may be the case is the growing number of long-term survivors of AIDS, some of whom no longer show any sign of the virus.

213

However, in the case of cancer, he mentions cases of "spontaneous remission," as reported by Dr. Lewis Thomas of Memorial Sloan-Kettering Cancer Center in a book called *Spontaneous Regression of Cancer* which discusses 176 patients. But the remissions occur among Christians and non-Christians, with and without prayer, and they represent a very small percentage of people with cancer who have been prayed for. He recounts various examples which illustrate the power of the mind to control the body.

This author views healing as a matter of external intervention, e.g., by medicine, doctors, or a supernatural power, rather than being the result of reliance on one's own internal resources. The people who were prayed for, but did not recover, may not have called upon their own natural healing power but relied upon an external intervention by a "healer," or the prayers of others.

A Course in Miracles. Foundation for Inner Peace, Glen Ellen, CA, 1975. A Text, Workbook with 365 lessons, and a Teacher's Guide. Described as "self-managed psychotherapy." Far more than "self help," the Course has been published in most languages and is in its sixteenth printing. Study groups can be found in every city and many towns—information about Oregon and Washington study groups is available from the Center for A Course in Miracles, 2518 S.E. 33rd Ave., Portland, OR 97202, (503) 235-1051, or from Miracle Distribution Center, 1141 E. Ash Ave., Fullerton, CA 92631 (for a list of national and international groups). A copy of the book (three volumes in one) may be ordered from either of these two centers for $25 softcover, $30 hardcover, or the three volumes published separately in hardback for $40, plus shipping and handling.

Cousins, Norman, *Anatomy of an Illness, as Perceived by the Patient: Reflections on Healing and Regeneration.* Cousins' account of his bout with a rare and serious blood disease. He checked himself out of the hospital and into a hotel room, where he watched video tapes of "Candid Camera" and laughed heartily for days. The resultant benefit to his body's ability to heal itself was quickly apparent, and he left the hotel cured of the disease which doctors had not been able to treat effectively.

Cousins, Norman, *The Healing Heart*. Avon Books, 1983. Cousins' account of his serious heart attack and his recovery, including his observations about needed changes in how the medical community "treats" heart attacks and other serious illnesses. Again, Cousins took a very active part in his own recovery.

DiOrio, Father Ralph A., *Called to Heal*. Doubleday, Image Books, 1984. As a priest, Fr. DiOrio has been called to a healing mission, of which he says the essence is: to give the love of Christ.

*Dossey, Larry, M.D., *Recovering the Soul: A Scientific and Spiritual Search*. Bantam Books, 1989. An exploration of the "nonlocal nature of our own minds, the rediscovery of our soul-like, nonlocal nature—the re-realization that we are eternal, infinite, and One." As a physician, Larry Dossey has often seen miraculous cures in his patients that cannot be explained by science and medicine. He refers to the wisdom of the West and the East to show how necessary is the synthesis and convergence of science, medicine, and spirituality. He describes in detail some fascinating and scientifically impeccable experiments from the Spindrift project in Salem, Oregon, in which rye seeds which were prayed for flourished more than those which were not, seeds which were prayed for *non-specifically* (i.e., "God's Will be done") did better than seeds which were prayed for with a specific purpose or intent, and seeds which received twice as much prayer flourished exactly twice as much as the others! A luminous, inspiring, thrilling and thought-provoking book

Drahos, Mary, *To Touch the Hem of His Garment: A True Story of Healing*. New York, Paulist Press, 1983. A book about divine healing, describing many personal experiences. The author was healed from infertility and from multiple sclerosis. She explains the relationship of divine healing to modern healing sciences and methods. She discusses the importance of "expectancy of recovery" (the secular equivalent of faith) in recovery from illness. The profoundly simple truth she finally discovered is this: In the final analysis, all genuine healing comes from God.

Foulks, Frances W. *Healing Everywhere.* Unity School of Christianity. A lovely little four-page pamphlet reminding us of what it takes to be healed. "To lie down in the stream of healing, to become submerged in the river of life, and to remain there, relaxed, expectant, is to feel the thrill of new life flowing into every cell of the body."

*Gawain, Shakti, *Creative Visualization.* Bantam Books, 1978. My personal favorite on visualization. A small book, but an inspired and inspiring guide to fulfillment of desires through the art of mental energy and affirmation.

Gendlin, Eugene T., *Focusing.* Bantam Books, 1978. Describes a new technique of self therapy that teaches you how to identify and change the way your personal problems concretely exist in your body. "Focusing guides you to the deepest level of awareness within your body, the only level where unresolved problems exist and can be changed." (See Ghandi, below, for an opposing point of view!)

Ghandi, Mahatma, *All Men Are Brothers.* Continuum, 1982. Autobiographical selections from his speeches and writings, reflecting his lifelong perpetual quest of truth. His life was rooted in India's religious tradition with its emphasis on a passionate search for truth, a profound reverence for life, the ideal of nonattachment, and the readiness to sacrifice all for the knowledge of God. From page 59: "God is not a person. . . God is the force. He is the essence of life. He is pure and undefiled consciousness. He is eternal. And yet, strangely enough, all are not able to derive either benefit from or shelter in the all-pervading life presence. Electricity is a powerful force. Not all can benefit from it. It can only be produced by following certain laws. It is a lifeless force. Man can utilize it if he labours hard enough to acquire the knowledge of its laws. The living force we call God can similarly be found if we know and follow His law leading to the discovery of Him in us." From Harijan, June 22, 1947: "To seek God one need not go on a pilgrimage or light lamps and burn incense before or anoint the image of the deity or paint it with red vermilion. For He resides in our hearts. If we could completely obliterate in us the consciousness of our physical body, we would see Him face to face."

Glassman, Judith. *The Cancer Survivors, and How They Did It*. Dial Press, 1984. A medical journalist investigates dozens of "hopeless" cases who have triumphed over cancer. Examines the methods they used, and comes to some surprising conclusions about the qualities that are necessary for survival. Extensive bibliography. Discusses "alternative treatments" for cancer.

Hellesby, O., *Prayer*. Augsberg Publishing House, 1931. A classic little book on prayer, written more than fifty years ago in Norway by a seminary professor who died in 1961. A practical and inspiring guide.

Helleberg, Marilyn Morgan. *Beyond TM: A Practical Guide to the Lost Tradition of Christian Meditation*. Paulist Press, 1980. Although some religions reject meditation as a pagan practice, this author reclaims the art of meditation as a deeply spiritual, Christian (though not religious) tradition related to prayer.

Hutschnecker, Arnold A., M.D., *The Will to Live*. Prentice Hall, 1951 and Simon & Schuster, Cornerstone Library, 1983. This classic has seen fifteen printings since 1951. A scientific interpretation of psychosomatic medicine, a very new concept at the time it was first published.

*Jampolsky, Gerald D., M.D., *Love is Letting Go of Fear*. Bantam Books, 1970. A primer on love and fear, the only two emotions there are.

*Jampolsky, Gerald D., M.D., *Teach Only Love: The Seven Principles of Attitudinal Healing*. Bantam Books, 1983. Jerry is the founder of the Center for Attitudinal Healing, a center in Tiburon, California for children with terminal illnesses, and their families. He applies the principles of the Course in Miracles to achieve healing of the spirit, and sometimes, healing of the body. Inspiring.

*Jampolsky, Gerald G., M.D., with Patricia Hopkins and William N. Thetford, Ph.D., *Goodbye to Guilt: Releasing Fear Through Forgiveness*. Bantam Books, 1985. A helpful discussion of a basic requirement in mental, spiritual, and physical healing: forgiveness.

Kubler-Ross, Elisabeth, *On Death and Dying*. This is the book in which Dr. Kubler-Ross formulated and described in detail the five stages of dying.

LeShan, Lawrence, *How to Meditate*. Little, Brown, 1974. Bantam Books, 1984. From reviewers: "A sound, discriminating manual for those put off elsewhere by cultist rhetoric. LeShan offers an authoritative, common-sense approach, compacting a wealth of information in a succinct beginner's guide to meditation." LeShan, a psychiatrist, teaches meditation as a way to reach "our fullest humanhood" (which some might call our divinity), our fullest sense of who we are and how we relate to each other and to the universe. Meditation is a technique found in every age and in every culture, in religious and secular philosophies, and in many forms. LeShan's guide is practical and specific, and provides exercises for you to use in tailoring meditation practices to your own needs and personality.

LeShan, Lawrence, *You Can Fight for Your Life: Emotional Factors in the Causation of Cancer*. Harcourt Brace Jovanovich, Jove Books, 1977. Identifies evidence that the mind and emotions may help make the body receptive to cancer. LeShan, a psychotherapist, carried out research with 71 patients who had been diagnosed as "terminal," to discover through therapy how to help the patients develop or regain their will to live. He found that the same factors that prevented cancer patients from fighting the disease often were linked to its development in the first place.

Lorde, Audre, *The Cancer Journals*. Spinsters, Ink, 1980. More than just a journal, poet and writer Lorde's startling perspective as a "post-mastectomy woman" offers comfort and a challenge. Refusing to wear a prosthesis ("Does Moshe Dayan wear a glass eye?"), she explores the meaning of breast amputation in a sexist society, and shares her grief, terror, courage, and passion for survival.

Marshall, Catherine, *The Helper*. Avon Books, 1978. Author guides us in relying on the Holy Spirit, the Helper, or Healer that Jesus left with us.

Merton, Thomas, *Contemplative Prayer*. Doubleday, Image Books, 1969. Written for younger monks, Merton tries to make ancient prayer and meditation principles applicable for today. He acknowledges the difficulty of meditating, and points out that the seemingly most labored and hard and seemingly unproductive meditation can cometimes prove to be the most successful after all (an experience often reported by meditators of all persuasions).

Mother Angelica, *Living Prayer*. Servant Books, 1985. Another useful book about the nature of prayer, including "dryness," and "prayer without ceasing."

*Peck, M. Scott, M.D., *The Road Less Traveled: A New Psychology of Love, Traditional Values, and Spiritual Growth*. Simon and Schuster, Touchstone Books, 1978. Interesting approach to therapy — he gives the four techniques of constructive problem-solving: delay of gratification, acceptance of responsibility, dedication to truth, and balancing. Major sections on Love, Growth and Religion, and a beautiful section on Grace. He discusses what he calls "scientific tunnel vision" (page 225).

*Pelletier, Kenneth R., *Mind as Healer, Mind as Slayer: A Holistic Approach to Preventing Stress Disorders*. Dell, Delta Books, 1977. The complex relationship between stress and disease, mind and body.

*Pepper, Curtis Bill, *We the Victors: The Inspiring Stories of People Who Conquered Cancer and How They Did It*. Doubleday, Signet Books, 1984. My favorite book for turning negative thinking to positive thinking! The author interviews and discusses cancer survivors who, for the most part, had been considered to be "terminal." He identifies the factors that seem to be present in every such case. I think the list is incomplete, but it sheds some light on the phenomenon of "spontaneous remission."

Porter, Garrett and Norris, Patricia A., *Why Me?: Harnessing the Healing Power of the Human Spirit*. Stillpoint Publishing, 1985. An inspiring account by a young boy who, with the help of his psychiatrist, healed himself of a malignant brain tumor through the power of visualization.

Samuels, Mike, M.D., and Samuels, Nancy, *Seeing With the Mind's Eye: The History, Techniques and Uses of Visualization*.

Sherman, Harold, *How to Picture What You Want*. Fawcett Gold Medial Books, 1978. Bestselling author on visualizing, imagery, and the power of the mind to control what happens to you. His basic law is this: *if an individual thinks* good *thoughts, he will eventually attract* good *things; if he thinks* bad *thoughts, he will ultimately attract* bad *things.*

Sherman, Harold, *The New TNT: The Miraculous Power Within You*. Prentice-Hall, 1966. More about the power of visualization, imaging, faith, words, ESP, healing.

*Siegel, Bernard, M.D., *Love, Medicine, and Miracles*. Harper and Row, 1986. A classic. Cancer patients, in particular, have found healing answers in this book by a surgeon who recognizes the connection between mind, spirit, and body. He has recognized that there are "exceptional patients" who seem to be able to tap their own internal healing powers and get well in spite of the worst prognoses.

*Simonton, Carl and Stephanie, *Getting Well Again*. Practical and useful techniques on how to fight cancer through the power of visualization and positive imagery. The Simontons are, respectively, a radiation oncologist and a psychologist, and used their techniques with cancer patients for whom all other treatments had failed, with some surprising successes. A cautionary note: wholesale acceptance of their findings can lead patients to feel guilty if they have a relapse, or don't get better. To quote Norman Cousins on that subject: "Sometimes physiology overwhelms psychology, and disease overtakes the best efforts of the patient to deal wih it through mental techniques." No guilt necessary, in other words. Positive visualization can enhance the effectiveness of chemotherapy and radiation therapy, and can enhance the well-being of the patient. In particular, it can give patients some control over what is happening to them. For another point of view on visualization, see Yogananda, below.

Stearns, Ann Kaiser, *Living Through Personal Crisis.* Ballantine Books, 1984. Recommended by Ann Landers as the best book to read in times of personal trauma. Emphasizes the importance of grieving, of not avoiding the pain, but going into it and experiencing it fully so that it may be released.

Weed, Joseph J., *Wisdom of the Mystic Masters.* Parker, Reward Books, 1968. A condensation of the ancient Rosicrucian wisdom that (as confirmed by modern brain specialists) we use less than five percent of our brain capacity. Everyone has the capacity to heal, through the power of psychic energy.

Yogananda, Paramahansa, *Scientific Healing Affirmations: Theory and Practice of Concentration.* Los Angeles, Self-Realization Fellowship Publishers, 1974. A small book describing the ancient art of healing through the scientific use of concentration and affirmations for healing inharmonies of the body, mind and soul through reason, will, feeling and prayer. This yogi first explains how affirmations heal, through the power of concentration, then gives a series of useful "affirmations" to use for various purposes. He reminds us that William James, in *Principles of Psychology*, points out that blisters can be healed by hypnosis.

About the Author

Judy Edwards Allen is on leave from Portland State University where she is an associate professor of education. She is the author of several textbooks in the area of educational technology.

She is chairperson of the board of directors for A Course In Miracles Center in Portland, Oregon, and facilitates study groups on healing.

Ordering Information

For additional copies of

> The Five Stages of ~~Death and Dying~~
> *Getting Well*
> by Judith E. Allen, or

> *Experiencing Guidance*
> by Frances Reed

Please enclose $14.95 per book, plus $2.00 shipping and handling for each book within the continental U.S.A.

International orders enclose $3.00 shipping and handling book rate (allow 8-10 weeks delivery) or $6.00 shipping and handling air mail.

Send orders to:

LifeTime Publishing
6914 SE 18th Ave.
Portland OR 97202-5723

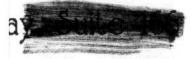

503-232-5699

Allow 2-4 weeks for delivery.

A Course in Miracles may be ordered from:
Center for A Course in Miracles
2518 S.E. 33rd Ave.
Portland, OR 97202
(503) 235-1051
for $25 (soft cover, three volumes in one) plus $3.00 for shipping and handling.